✅ Y0-BDA-926

Looking Beyond the Entry Issue:
Implications for Education and Service

Pub. No. 41-2173

WY
21.1
.L66
1986

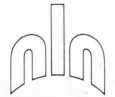

National League for Nursing • New York

Manufactured in the United States of America.

Contents

PART III: SERVICE ISSUES

APPENDIXES

Contributors

Connie R. Curran, EdD, RN, FAAN, is Vice President, American Hospital Association, Chicago, Illinois.

Vivien DeBack, PhD, RN, is Director, National Commission on Nursing Implementation Project, Milwaukee, Wisconsin.

Sylvia Edge, MA, RN is Director of Council Affairs, Council of Associate Degree Programs, National League for Nursing, New York, New York.

Shirley H. Fondiller, EdD, RN, is Executive Director, Mid-Atlantic Regional Nursing Association, New York, New York.

Sylvia E. Hart, PhD, RN, is Dean and Professor, College of Nursing, University of Tennessee, Knoxville.

Denise Hartung, MSN, RN, is head nurse in surgery, Strong Memorial Hospital, University of Rochester Medical Center, Rochester, New York.

Pamela J. Maraldo, PhD, RN, is Executive Director, National League for Nursing, New York, New York.

Clair E. Martin, PhD, RN, is Dean and Professor, Nell Hodgson Woodruff School of Nursing, Emory University, Atlanta, Georgia.

Carl Miller, DNSc, RN, is Professor and Chairman, Level IV, School of Nursing, University of Alabama at Birmingham.

Neale Miller, MSN, RN, is Program Director, Education, Titling, and Licensure, Division of Nursing, American Hospital Association, Chicago, Illinois.

Tim Porter-O'Grady, EdD, RN, is President, Affiliated Dynamics, Norcross, Georgia.

Theresa G. Sharp, EdD, RN, is Associate Professor, College of Nursing, University of Tennessee, Knoxville.

Foreword

Pamela J. Maraldo

The intense emotionalism surrounding the entry-into-practice issue and all its implications is, at least in part, rooted in fears that stem from a lack of information. Many in the nursing community and in other parts of the health care system harbor misconceptions about national organizations' positions on the issues related to titling and licensure, about opportunities for educational mobility, and about the prospects for implementing a titling and licensure position in the 50 states. Therefore, amidst the current strident debate over titling and licensure in the nursing and larger health care community, it behooves us to examine carefully the national trends and issues related to the entire titling and licensure arena.

This collection of works seeks to shed light on these questions in hopes of generating greater informed debate on all sides of the titling and licensure issue. The work begins with the historical and sociological origins of the age-old entry dilemma for nursing. Then it moves to a particularly enlightening discussion of the issues and options found in the current system of nursing education, dispelling myths about educational mobility, and explaining existing routes for educational advancement and the reasons for them. The latest information on the National Commission on Nursing Implementation Project and what it seeks to accomplish will enlighten readers about the thinking of organized nursing regarding the differences that exist in the two levels of practice as they were conceptualized, and the limits of these original conceptualizations.

The last section of the book takes a hard look at the anticipated short-term impact of titling and licensure changes in the workplace. The longer-term problems associated with recruiting qualified applicants into nursing in the future are also examined.

In the final analysis, it is most important for all of us to keep in mind that credentialing mechanisms exist primarily for societal reasons: to protect the public against harmful forces and incidents, whether it be protecting government agencies against fraud and abuse, assisting students to identify acceptable institutions, making education more responsive to students' and society's needs, or offsetting the dangers of government control of education. Licensure laws in particular are concerned with the public safety, and licensure differs from the other two credentialing mechanisms (accreditation and certification) in that it is controlled and administered as a governmental function. Licensure is a prerogative of the state and therefore is regulated through nurse practice acts. It is also distinct from accreditation and certification in that it examines the individual for attainment of the *minimum* degree of competency necessary to ensure the public health, safety, and welfare. Indeed, it is essentially a method of protecting the public from unsafe, incompetent practitioners.

Licensure laws originated at the end of the nineteenth century because of professional groups' struggles to maintain their own identity against corporate dominance and control. Consequently, the movement was not restricted to professionals, but included plumbers, barbers, horseshoers, pharmacists, embalmers, and sundry other groups that sought and were granted licensure protection.

Accreditation and certification, as well as licensure, were originally conceived and instituted for the sake of protecting the public and ensuring quality care to the public. Yet, several experts believe that these original purposes have been thwarted. These critics accuse licensure boards of being self-seeking, self-serving, self-perpetuating, monopolistic, and oriented toward professional rather than consumer interests. Others maintain the view that nursing boards—as well as other licensure boards—are effective and necessary consumer watchdogs, and without them the public safety would surely be placed in jeopardy. Still others concede that licensure is a political tool and, as such, professional use of licensure statutes to generate professional control not only is not a bad thing but is, in fact, desirable.

Viewed in this light, licensure gives professions greater control over standards of care delivered and a greater say as to who can and cannot become the new members of their ranks. Having a greater voice over who enters the profession, how new members are educated, and who achieves excellence affords professionals the opportunity to exercise their own world views and values in a system of competing interests. In fact, credentialing can be and is considered a political issue: credentialing is a process of governance over the American educational-professional system. Even though credentialing agencies—private or public—are holders of a public trust, they are governed by individuals with private interests and limited resources, and that makes credentialing, in the final analysis, a political matter. Individuals are not usually willing to set aside their private affairs for the sake of a collective good. There is therefore a need for incentives in these matters, and licensure may be considered to be one such incentive to gain control over individual practitioners for the collective good so that the profession can regulate itself, in the public's as well as its own best interests.

As many nursing leaders and policymakers have emphasized, it is imperative that nurses approach the political arena with a unified, cohesive strategy that would prevent other interest groups from dictating the standards of nursing practice or evaluating nursing practice. In credentialing arenas, as in other political arenas, nursing's inability to generate strong collective organization reflects a fundamental weakness in our professional fabric that is rooted in a lack of strength in common shared interests.

In spite of competing values and loyalties, internal conflicts, and class differences that have prevented understanding and articulation of common interests, nursing must continually strengthen and revitalize itself and strive to devote its efforts, energies, and other resources to looking out for the health needs of the public. If we do not, we will have little influence over this, our rightful domain.

Self-regulation is our right and, indeed, our responsibility for the public's sake and for nursing's own sake. That is not to say that nursing or any other profession should feather its own nest and be concerned only with self-serving interests. If nursing does not have sufficient confidence in its own abilities and its own perspective, credentialing mechanisms will not assist in producing the kind of practitioners that the public needs and deserves. This collection of works will make a contribution toward assisting nursing in this effort.

PART I

Perspectives on the Problem

CHAPTER 1

Licensure and Titling in Nursing and Society: A Historical Perspective

Shirley H. Fondiller

Licensure is the oldest of credentialing mechanisms for regulating the practice of a profession or occupation to protect the health, safety, and welfare of the public. The authority to grant licensure is conferred by the fourteenth amendment to the Constitution of the United States, which gives police power to the states. This power, designed to police human activities involving the safety, life, morals, and health of the nation's people, is the source of authority for all laws regulating trades, businesses, and occupations.

In 1971, the U.S. Department of Health, Education, and Welfare defined licensure as "the process by which an agency of government grants permission to an individual to engage in a given occupation upon finding that the applicant has attained the minimal degree of competency necessary to ensure that the public health, safety, and welfare will be protected" (Office of the Assistant Secretary for Health and Scientific Affairs, 1971). When the report of the American Nurses' Association's study of credentialing in nursing was released in 1979, the study committee expanded the definition to include a reference to titling:

> Licensing is a process by which an agency of state government grants permission to individuals accountable for the practice of a profession to engage in the practice of that profession

3

and prohibits all others from legally doing so. It permits use
of a particular title. Its purpose is to protect the public by
ensuring a minimum level of professional competence [p. 64].

Some authorities characterize the licensure of professions and
occupations as a "patchwork quilt," with similarities as well as
differences in the laws within states as well as among them. In
1952, the U.S. Supreme Court noted that the rise of regulatory
agencies in the nation represented the most significant legal trend
of the twentieth century. It pointed out that more values have
been influenced by the decisions of these agencies than by "those
of all the courts, review of administrative decisions apart" (*F.T.C. v.
Ruberoid Co.*, 1952).

Acquiring an understanding of the regulatory process is essential to any discussion of the concept of licensure. The impact of
agencies involved had its beginnings with the Act of July 31, 1789,
which established the first federal agency to estimate duties pay-
able on imports as well as other related duties (Waddle, 1979).
Since that time, Congress, state, and local governments have passed
legislation to regulate different activities, and to establish agencies
to administer the laws. Through the years, the increasing complexity of society and governments has created a circular pattern
in which services and programs are sought, laws and regulations
are established, and then criticism is usually imposed on the regulatory process.

During the late 1960s and into the 1970s, the American people
had increasing exposure to the regulatory system because of its
visibility in the political arena in forums ranging from local councils to the Presidential campaign. Waddle (1979) has identified
several concerns relating to regulation: (1) the effect on competition, (2) the cost to the consumer through increased charges for
services and products, (3) control of the regulatory agency by the
industry being regulated, (4) the difficulty of changing regulatory
measures once they are established, and (5) the fact that the industry itself, rather than the public, usually determines the regulation.

Although licensure has been around for a long time, in recent
years it has assumed more prominence, in particular among the
health care disciplines. Contributing factors have included the rise
of new categories of health workers, increased costs of health
care, and the maldistribution of health care workers. The licensure
of nurses, which made its appearance in the early twentieth century, has become an integral part of the American tradition. Its

history has been closely linked to the professional associations and their efforts to protect the public through the monitoring and furthering of nursing education standards.

EVOLUTION OF LICENSURE

The training and licensing of individuals in the professions can be traced to the universities of the Middle Ages, when a degree represented a certificate of competence, particularly in medicine and law. During that period, the guilds—which later evolved into professional bodies—also offered training to their members that conferred exclusive rights of practice. When the guilds began to phase out, the state took over the training and licensing responsibilities. Rather then establish new training agencies, however, it depended on the universities and other institutions of higher learning to provide the necessary educational requirements.

When European settlers came to the New World in the early seventeenth century, they brought all the traditions, values, and ideas inherent in their earlier life styles. In colonial America, university training became a prerogative of the wealthy, whereas others who wished to prepare for the professions learned through an apprentice-type system. The latter approach produced many incompetent physicians and lawyers. In 1639, the first attempt by government to regulate the practice of medicine was instituted by the state of Virginia, with similar statutes enacted in Massachusetts in 1649 and New York in 1665. Impetus for the laws came from public complaints and the need to distinguish between charges issued against persons with university training and those with apprenticeship training.

A number of medical practice acts appeared between 1700 and 1800, with the first comprehensive legislation passed by New Jersey. The laws provided that the regulation of medicine be placed under a state board of examiners composed of all lay members (Waddle, 1979). By the turn of the nineteenth century, 13 of the 16 existing states had adopted laws giving medical societies the authority to examine and license. The trend to upgrade standards in the medical profession, however, was short-lived, and by the time of the Civil War, attempts to strip the societies of their licensing power had succeeded. The result was that not one state had an effective licensing system. Furthermore, any person who wanted to perform an act of healing could do so.

In the decade following the war, public outrage accompanied

by outcries of fraud and incompetence cleared the path for reform in medical practice. Through the efforts of local, state, and national associations or societies, codes of ethics were developed and enforced and standards of competence established. These groups also worked for the passage of the necessary legislation.

The establishment of a licensure system connoted legal approval of ethical codes of the associations, which also stipulated that a legal register be instituted to record qualified practitioners. The system gave a stamp of approval as well as status to the medical profession and its members. In addition, the demand for state control over licensing carried some weight for the professional associations in their efforts to seek representation on the licensing agencies.

Between 1873 and 1900, medical boards were formed in every state in the Union. Their success in raising standards was a timely development for the nursing profession just getting organized around that same period. Eventually, when nursing proposed its own legislation for the registration of nurses, it was patterned after the laws establishing the state board of medical examiners (Shannon, 1975).

HISTORY OF NURSING LICENSURE

It was through the work of Florence Nightingale that nursing first achieved recognition of its occupational status. Her principal contribution, however, was to clarify for the public not so much what nursing was but rather what it was not. She eliminated those aspects relating to charitable obligation, religious requirement, and domestic duty. She described nursing as a means of obtaining a livelihood through practice based on a sound scientific foundation.

Nightingale's views on nursing licensure or state board examinations differed markedly from those of nursing leaders in her own country and in the United States. She believed that the educational program should be of such quality that it would not be necessary for the individual to acquire approval from the government. "We do not give the woman a printed certificate," she wrote, "but simply enter the names of all certified nurses in the register as such. This was done to prevent them, in the event of misconduct, from using their certification improperly" (Nightingale, 1867, p. 2).

Proponents of the registration movement in Great Britain, who were waging a long and arduous battle for registration, saw this mechanism as the first step toward eliminating unqualified or incompetent nurses. Their most staunch advocate, Ethel Bedford-Fenwick (1903), identified the opposing position as a conservative attempt to maintain the status quo. She attributed the many defeats encountered to the lack of public support, especially from the privileged class. When Bedford-Fenwick acquired the *Nursing Record* (later called the *British Journal of Nursing*) in the early 1890s, she used the journal to further the registration cause.

In 1892, she visited the United States and met with nursing leaders to arrange a Nursing Section in conjunction with the International Congress of Charities, Correction, and Philanthropy to be held during the Chicago World's Fair the following year. Educational and registration issues were a prime concern at the historic Congress, which spawned nursing's first professional organization in the United States—the American Society of Superintendents of Training Schools for Nursing (renamed the National League of Nursing Education, or NLNE, in 1912).

From its inception, the society made its principal objective the establishment and maintenance of a universal standard of training. Its members, an elite group within the profession, also recognized the importance of an organizational arrangement to accommodate the needs of practicing nurses. Their efforts led to the founding of another national association in 1896 known as the Nurses' Associated Alumnae of the United States and Canada. The Alumnae Association (it became the American Nurses' Association—ANA—in 1914) cited as its purpose to "strengthen the union of existing nursing organizations, to elevate nursing education, and to promote ethical standards in all relations of the nursing profession" (Piemonte, 1976).

With the establishment of training schools for nurses, beginning in 1873 at Bellevue Hospital, New Haven Hospital, and Massachusetts General Hospital, a rapid proliferation began to occur which resulted in 432 schools by 1900. However, their lack of uniformity in requirements and standards as well as the controls imposed by external forces caused nursing leaders some concern. Training programs ranged from six months to two years, with each school setting its own standards. Service needs of the hospital took priority over the educational needs of the students. Since a graduate of any school could call herself a "trained nurse," the public was unable to differentiate the safe from the unsafe practitioner (Connors, 1967).

Between 1898 and 1902, momentum for registration was gaining with the formation of state nurses' associations. In 1900, the newly launched *American Journal of Nursing* became a powerful voice for the profession with the frequent proregistration editorials of Sophie Palmer. At the Third International Congress of Nurses in Buffalo, New York, in 1901, Ethel Bedford-Fenwick proclaimed the need for a system of registration to be automatically regulated by nursing and to guarantee the qualifications of nurses (Birnbach, 1982, p. 48).

On March 3, 1903, the licensing of nurses in America became a reality when North Carolina became the first state to enact legislation of this type. By 1913, 20 states had similar laws, and all states had them by 1923. No attempt was made to define and control the practice of nursing. The laws aimed only to recognize those practitioners who had met the standards of training set by the state licensing board and therefore were entitled to call themselves registered nurses. Until 1947, the laws controlled practitioners and titles but not the practice itself. Thus, they were called *nurse* practice acts rather than *nursing* practice acts—the name by which they later came to be known (Anderson, 1950, p. 36).

From the outset, titling was a concern of state nurses' associations in promoting legislation for nurses' licensure. In the early 1890s, British advocates of registration had adopted the title of "registered nurse." American leaders believed that the incorporation of a universal title into the bill in each state would minimize confusion, enhance conformity, and facilitate the movement of nurses from one state to another (Dock, 1902). In the fall of 1902, the New York State Nurses' Association queried its membership by mail about an appropriate title and offered the choices of graduate nurse, certified nurse, trained nurse, registered graduate nurse, or registered nurse. At the next meeting, the majority of association members voted on the title of registered nurse (Birnbach, 1982, p. 74). When North Carolina's nurse licensure law was passed, it identified the licensed practitioner as registered nurse.

Since the state laws stipulated that nurses be licensed to practice, the term *licensure* has become widely accepted. At the time of the early statutes, however, *registration* was the term universally applied to the movement, except in rare cases (Birnbach, 1982, p. 4). In 1979, the ANA Study Committee on Credentialing defined registration as

> a process by which qualified individuals are listed on an official register maintained by a government or non-governmental agency. It enables such persons to use a particular title and

attests to employing agencies and individuals that minimum qualifications have been met and maintained [American Nurses' Association, 1979, p. 66].

As state nurses' associations began to organize in the nation, nurse licensure acts were enacted. However, unlike the medical licensure laws, which were originally established to eliminate quackery, comparable legislation for nurses was not intended to correct abuses of independent practice. Its purpose was to protect both the nurse and the public from unqualified and unethical practitioners. Furthermore, several states passed permissive nurse practice acts that required the licensing of nurses only if they wished to enjoy the rights and privileges provided by licensure. Under these acts, others could practice nursing provided that they did not represent themselves as registered nurses or use other controlled titles and abbreviations. Mandatory licensure, on the other hand, gave a precise definition of a licensed nurse using the words "all who nurse for hire," and prevented unauthorized persons from practicing nursing (Anderson, 1950, p. 4). Yet, even in states with mandatory licensure, many of the laws contained exemptions.

Regardless of the ambiguity and looseness of the registration laws, they led to some reforms in nursing education. Entrance standards of training schools were upgraded from one year of high school preparation to four. Nursing courses in schools improved in quality, and more subjects were added to the curriculum. Also, new teaching equipment was introduced, along with better housing for students. In addition, nurses took more interest in seeking postgraduate courses. Another benefit of the registration laws was their impact on moving nursing into the higher education system. By 1916, a total of 16 colleges and universities maintained schools, departments, or courses in nursing education.

Because of the unevenness in the provisions of nursing statutes among the states, a nurse registered in one state having lower standards would be prevented from practicing in another state with higher standards. As far back as 1904, Nutting identified this problem and suggested the establishment of a central examining board, advisory board, or board of control to obtain uniformity. Many years later, Anderson (1950) wrote: "although the desires of many for uniform nursing practice acts in all the states must remain a Utopian dream, nevertheless, serious efforts are being made to work out reasonable solutions on a voluntary basis" (p. 14). Some of the activities exerting the greatest influence in that direction included the annual state board conference sponsored jointly by the American Nurses' Association and the National League of Nursing Education; the ANA Bureau of State Board of Examiners formed in 1943; and the national state board test pool operated for several years by the NLNE's Department of Measurement and Guidance.

LICENSING BOARDS AND TESTING

Licensing boards were created as administrative agencies for implementing an occupation or profession's practice acts as specified in the statutes enacted by the respective state legislatures. According to the early laws, board members were elected by members of their professional association. In time, however, this system changed to provide for the appointment of board members by a state official (usually the governor), who obtained a list of names proposed by the professional association.

In the 1970s a trend developed to include one or more public members on the licensing boards, and public officials have been appointed to serve in some states. A shared responsibility between the public and occupational or professional licensing board can be viewed as a positive step toward ensuring greater accountability for the future.

Historically, as state boards of nursing examiners developed, they began to see a need for some kind of mechanism to discuss mutual needs and increasing concerns. In 1912, at a special conference on state registration laws, held during the ANA convention, the participants voted to form a committee that would arrange an annual conference for individuals involved with state boards of nursing (Malone, Fondiller, and Heidorn, 1983). As part of ANA's structure, the new committee worked to promote uniform standards, improve methods and procedures of member boards, and approve basic nursing education programs that prepared nurses for licensure.

Boards of nursing also worked closely with NLNE which, in June 1933, accepted the responsibility for advisory services to the state boards of nurse examiners in all education matters, including the examination. Through its Committee on Education, NLNE formed a subcommittee on state board examination problems. In 1937, the League published an important document, *A Curriculum Guide for Schools of Nursing*, which had implications for the state boards in that it focused attention on the objective evaluation of the nursing student. Two years later, the organization initiated the first testing service through its Committee on Nursing Tests.

Under the leadership of Isabel Stewart as chair and R. Louise McManus as secretary, the committee developed a battery of tests—the Pre-Nursing and Guidance Test Battery—for use by faculties of state-approved schools of nursing in selecting and placing students. In May 1941, the first experimental prenursing examinations were successfully administered, and they were later extended to other states on request. The introduction of nursing tests came at a time when the nation was entering World War II and nursing schools needed to recruit qualified students. Nurse examiners also had to deal with pressures to hasten licensing and to schedule examinations more frequently.

In December 1942 at an emergency conference called by NLNE's Committee on State Board Problems, state board examiners suggested a pooling of tests, in which each state would prepare machine-scoreable examinations in only one or two subjects that would provide a reservoir of tests or test items (Malone, Fondiller, and Heidorn, 1983). With approval from NLNE's Board of Directors, the Committee on Nursing Tests assumed the responsibility for operating a pool of licensing tests for interested states.

Following NLNE's decision to move ahead in this direction, a number of problems arose. Many states found it difficult to provide promptly any objective-type tests for use by the pool. Furthermore, committee staff were unable to adapt the test items, finding insufficient content to develop a machine-scoreable examination of nursing competence in each subject on the test. To resolve the situation, the Committee on Nursing Tests decided to draft complete tests in each subject, using as a guide the blueprint of a test of nursing competency in medical nursing. In January 1944, when the first series of the State Board Test Pool Examination (SBTPE) for professional nursing licensure was released, it consisted of 13 tests used in total or in part by 22 states and the District of Columbia. Six years later, every state in the nation and some provinces in Canada were using the SBTPE. Over 27,000 candidates for RN licensure were tested, compared with 8,595 in 1944 (Malone Fondiller, and Heidorn, 1983).

Following the consolidation of the national nursing organizations in 1952, the new National League for Nursing, through its Evaluation and Guidance Service, continued with the state board activities formerly undertaken by the NLNE. Boards of nursing recommended nurse educators who were specialists in each area of the examination to work with the test development staff.

Through the years, state licensing boards also maintained a close relationship with the American Nurses' Association. During the early forties, members of the Conference of State Boards of

Nurse Examiners recognized the need for a national clearinghouse that could provide them with information. Thus, the ANA Bureau of State Boards of Nursing came into existence in 1943, with its work guided by a committee of the organization. When the bureau became established in ANA's bylaws, its functions were described as follows: (1) to collect and disseminate data regarding state board statistics, activities, and practices; (2) to devise methods and procedures for bringing about desirable and reasonable uniformity in relation to standards, regulations, examinations, and records; (3) to carry out studies and supply the necessary field service; and (4) to cooperate with nursing organizations in forwarding the objectives of organized nursing (Malone, Fondiller, and Heidorn, p. 9).

In 1947, ANA appointed a committee to function under the Bureau of State Boards of Nurse Examiners. Originally consisting of nurse representatives from each state board, the committee later expanded to include representatives of NLNE and the Association for Collegiate Schools of Nursing as well as ANA staff. In 1961, the ANA Committee of State Boards of Nursing appointed a subcommittee to explore the parent committee's operations, particularly how it functioned within the professional association. As a result, a Council of State Boards of Nursing was proposed in lieu of the committee.

ANA's participation in the state board examination was initiated in 1954 with the appointment of a Blueprint Committee, whose chief function was to develop core test plans for the tests in each series of the examination for registered nurse licensure and practical nurse licensure. Item writers selected by a subcommittee worked with NLN's test service staff to develop test questions for the initial drafts of the licensure examination. Each jurisdiction then was able to participate in the development of questions. The responsibility for the content of each examination ultimately rested with the Blueprint Committee.

When annual licensure examinations were initiated in 1968, the procedure for developing test items underwent some change. New items were placed in item reservoirs rather than being written for the next test to be administered. Examinations for the future were selected from reservoirs of test items that had complete documentation and item analysis data on file. In time, candidates for the nurse licensure examination increased substantially, and by 1978, 118,277 RN candidates and 54,521 PN candidates were tested (Malone, Fondiller, and Heidorn, 1983, p. 11).

The year 1978 was highly significant because it also marked the dissolution of the ANA Council of State Boards of Nursing. In its place, a new organization was launched called the National Council of State Boards of Nursing. Questions had been raised about the appropriateness of a Council of State Boards of Nursing within the professional association, and after years of study, its members voted to establish a freestanding organization of state boards of nursing. Although many of the procedures for developing the licensure examination were continued, some major changes occurred under the National Council. Within a few years, the licensure examination underwent a major revision in format, and a new agency other than the National League for Nursing was selected to develop the state board test pool examination. In the early 1980s, the name of the test was changed to the National Council Licensing Examination (NCLEX), and a criterion-referenced scoring system was instituted.

THE QUESTION OF TITLING

To the American public, titles such as registered nurse and licensed practical nurse have become familiar terminology. Although consumers may not always be able to describe the preparation and practice of the two types of nurses, they are generally aware that differences exist. Practical nurses and registered nurses alike have clung tenaciously to their titles as marks of identity that have long characterized their respective involvements in the health care field.

The title of practical nurse came under serious scrutiny in the late 1940s when the NLNE Board of Directors at a meeting in Cleveland suggested that a different name might project a more favorable image for recruitment purposes (National League for Nursing Education, 1949). Some board members believed that a new designation such as nursing technician would eliminate any housekeeping connotation associated with the trained practical nurse. Others responded unfavorably, however, pointing out that the NLNE Committee on Practical Nurse Education and the U.S. Office of Education were planning to issue a publication on the practical nursing curriculum and strongly opposed any change in name.

In 1950, the Joint Committee on Practical Nurses and Auxiliary Workers[1] presented the NLNE board with its reasons for retaining

---

[1] The committee consisted of representatives of the American Nurses' Association, National League of Nursing Education, National Organization for Public Health Nursing, Association of Collegiate Schools of Nursing, National Association of Colored Graduate Nurses, and the National Organization for Practical Nurse Education

the title of practical nurse in lieu of nursing technician (National League for Nursing Education, 1950):

1. Practical nurses themselves should have an opportunity to discuss any title change proposed for the group.
2. The word "technician" implies interest in techniques only.
3. The title "practical nurse" was only recently approved by all nursing organizations and the public is just beginning to know what is meant by trained practical nurses. A change would add to existing confusion over a variety of titles now in use.
4. All recent and pending legislation has used the title "licensed practical nurse."
5. The new national association used the title of "licensed practical nurse."

Although no further attempt was made for some years to change the practical nurse title, the term nursing technician assumed further significance in the early 1950s when Mildred Montag, in an innovative study, proposed a new type of technical nursing preparation. Its purpose, Montag (1951) stated, was to "plan a program for the preparation of the nurse with predominantly technical functions and to propose a program for the preparation of nurse personnel for faculty positions in these programs" (p. 9). In her study, she projected a curriculum of two academic years in length, but with the understanding that it would be tried out and studied carefully.

Aware that safety of the public should be the main consideration of licensing, Montag (1951) stressed one licensure for nurses:

> The nursing profession should support a comprehensive accrediting program for all schools of nursing, carry on a positive program of information so the public may be informed and work for an inclusive mandatory licensing system [p. 82].

Some years later, Montag reconsidered her position on licensure and recommended two discrete licenses for nursing—one for the baccalaureate-prepared nurse, the other for the associate degree nurse. In the beginning, she stated, there were not enough professionally prepared (baccalaureate) practitioners. "We had to prove that the A.D. graduate could pass a licensing exam that was really geared to the diploma graduate" (quoted in Fondiller, 1976).

In developing her concept of a new worker in nursing, Montag noted that it was appropriate to call one skilled in the techniques of nursing a technician. She also believed that the term nursing technician would not satisfy forever; in time, this person became known as the associate degree nurse.

Anderson (1966), commenting about professional and technical nursing preparation, pointed to the numerous discussions in the nursing literature about the merits and contributions of two competently prepared nurses having complementary roles. She cited two important problems in achieving this goal:

> The first will be one of terminology or titles for these nurses. The second will be whether nursing is willing or able to plan and bring about a merging of all existing nurses into the appropriate categories, and education for nursing into professional and technical only. Corollary problems flowing out of such action will be of two kinds. The first will be one of terminology or titles for achieving understandable competent nursing care for the people of our country . . . [p. 283].

The late 1960s marked the beginning of a new era in American nursing with the profession's strong push for clinical specialization. Another major development was the evolving role of the nurse practitioner, a new type of health professional whose work in primary care differed markedly from the traditional model. Perhaps no other group has been more diligently studied than nurse practitioners in relation to their titles, roles, and perceptions.

In 1971, the U.S. Department of Health, Education, and Welfare issued a report entitled *Extending the Scope of Nursing Practice*, which represented the joint efforts of nursing, medicine, hospital administration, and other health disciplines to define problems in health care and make recommendations for enlarging the scope of nursing practice. Although the report noted that the implementation of expanded roles for nurses would require some legal evaluation, it did not believe that state licensure would create any difficulty. It urged that more attention be paid to the "commonality of nursing licensure and certification and to the development and acceptance of a model law of nursing practice suitable for national application throughout the state." In the ensuing years, significant changes occurred in legal regulation of the practice of nurse practitioners through changes in nursing practice acts, changes in health insurance laws, and the promulgation of rules and regulations to support the advanced practice of nursing.

A breakthrough for the profession came in the middle seventies when the New York State Nurses' Association obtained passage of a revised nursing practice act that distinguished between nursing practice and medical practice and acknowledged nursing as an autonomous profession. Nursing was defined as "diagnosing and treating human responses to actual or potential health problems through such means as case finding, health teaching, and counseling" (quoted in Kalisch & Kalisch, 1978, p. 666). The new law was an important event because it provided for the first time a definition establishing statutory authority for the practice of nursing.

PROPOSALS FOR REFORM

Although some attempts have been made to strengthen state practice acts, the profession still has a long way to go in achieving uniformity of standards. These acts are among the few licensing laws for professions and occupations that do not require graduation from a nationally accredited school or educational program as a prerequisite for the licensure examination. It should be noted that the terms "approval" and "accreditation," frequently used interchangeably at the state level, are not synonymous. The term approval, which appears in most nursing practice acts, means a mechanism utilized by a governmental agency. Accreditation, on the other hand, applies to standards that are higher than the minimum standards set by the governmental agency. Accrediting agencies require that the school or program be approved by the state before applying for accreditation.

The parameters of nursing practice in many states continue to be ill-defined. Professionals are eligible to use the title registered nurse, whereas assisting personnel are called licensed practical nurses or licensed vocational nurses. The new designation of associate or associate nurse may add more confusion to an already chaotic situation. Furthermore, the laws that grant credentials to beginning practitioners in some states also control advanced or specialty practice. A number of jurisdictions monitor the activities of untrained nursing assistants.

During the 1970s, a move was underway by several nursing specialty organizations to explore licensure for specialty practitioners in addition to the RN licensure credential. Critics of these efforts have decried them as contrary to the basic principles of licensure whose aim initially is to show that the individual has met certain requirements for minimal competency as established by state law (Waddle, 1979, p. 3). Traditionally, specialty practice has been accorded certification by a professional association, which recognizes that additional qualifications have been met.

The Study of Credentialing in Nursing (American Nurses' Association, 1979) cited four major weaknesses existing in licensing practices that must be considered in planning any change: (1) the lack of a defined scope of practice for licensure; (2) dependence on the state boards of nursing approval of schools for assuring qualified clinical practitioners; (3) the paucity of lay representatives on boards of nursing; and (4) the lack of an effective monitoring system for individual accountability.

One of the more significant recommendations of the study related to the type of nursing practitioner who should be licensed. It was the study committee's belief that "professional nurses (defined by the professional society and state law), as the persons accountable for the *entire scope of nursing practice*, be the only licensed members of the occupation" (p. 65). Assisting nursing personnel (to be defined and titled by the professional society) should be registered by a national, nongovernmental agency, using publicly announced criteria and evaluation procedures. Those individuals, who perform specific functions necessary to the practice of nursing but do not engage in the full scope of practice, will need to reregister for continued competency, since this type of practice changes rapidly. As the study committee pointed out, national rather than state registration would permit greater mobility for the individual in responding to personal and public needs. It also would offer better coordination and permit flexibility for change.

A discussion of licensure and titling would be incomplete without some recognition of the social, political, and legal factors that influence the system. Certainly, enlightened American consumers with their increasing distrust of the government and the regulatory process have intensified the need to strengthen licensing procedures. If the nursing profession is genuine in its pledge to protect the health and welfare of the public it serves, then nurses must move forward and collectively institute the necessary reforms.

REFERENCES

American Nurses' Association. (1979). *The study of credentialing in nursing: A new approach: Vol. 1. The report of the committee.* Kansas City, MO: American Nurses' Association.

Anderson, B. (1950). *The facilitation of interstate movement of registered nurses.* Philadelphia: J. B. Lippincott Co.

Anderson, B. (1966). *Nursing education in community junior colleges.* Philadelphia: J. B. Lippincott Co.

Bedford-Fenwick, E. (1903). Letter to the superintendents at Detroit, Official reports of societies. *American Journal of Nursing, 3*(2), 126–128.

Birnbach, N. (1982). *The genesis of the nurse registration movement in the United States, 1893–1903.* Unpublished doctoral dissertation, Teachers College, Columbia University.

Connors, H. V. (1967, Winter). Laws regulating the practice of nursing. In *State Government.* Lexington, KY: Council of State Governments.

Dock, L. (1902, December). Letter to the Editor. *American Journal of Nursing, 2,* 240–241.

F.T.C. v. Ruberoid Co., 343 U.S. 470, 487, 72S. Ct. 800, 810, 1952.

Fondiller, S. (1983). *The entry dilemma: The National League for Nursing and the Higher Education Movement, 1952–1972.* New York: National League for Nursing.

Fondiller, S. (1976, May 5). Entry into professional practice—NYSNA proposal at issue. *American Nurse, 9,* 7.

Kalisch, P., & Kalisch, B. (1978). *The advance of American nursing.* Boston: Little, Brown & Co., 666.

Malone, G., Fondiller, S., & Heidorn, D. (1983). *From an idea to an organization.* Chicago: National Council of State Boards of Nursing.

Montag, M. (1951). *The education of nursing technicians.* New York: G. Putnam's Sons.

National League for Nursing Education. (1949). *Minutes, NLNE Board of Directors, April 28–30, 1949.* National League for Nursing Archives, New York.

National League for Nursing Education. (1950). *Minutes, NLNE Board of Directors, January 23–25, 1950.* National League for Nursing Archives, New York.

Nightingale, F. (1867). Suggestions for the improvement of the nursing service of hospitals and on the method of training nurses for the sick poor. Reprinted from *Blue Book, Report on Cubic Space in Metropolitan Workhouses.*

Nutting, A. (1904, July). State reciprocity. *American Journal of Nursing, 4,* 781–782.

Office of the Assistant Secretary for Health and Scientific Affairs. (1971). *Report on licensure and related health personnel credentialing* (Publication No. (HMS) 72-11). Washington, DC: Department of Health, Education, & Welfare.

Piemonte, R. V. (1976). *A history of the National League of Nursing Education 1912–1932: Great awakening in nursing education.* Doctoral dissertation,

Teachers College, Columbia University. Available from University Microfilms International.

Shannon, M. L. (1975, August). Our first four licensure laws. *American Journal of Nursing, 75*(8), 1329.

U.S. Department of Health, Education, and Welfare (1971). *Extending the scope of nursing practice: Report of the secretary's committee to study the extended roles for nurses.* Washington, DC: U.S. Government Printing Office.

Waddle, F. (1979). Licensure: Achievements and limitation. In American Nurses' Association, *The study of credentialing in nursing: A new approach: Vol. 2. Staff working papers.* Kansas City, MO: American Nurses' Association.

CHAPTER 2

A Sociological Perspective on Professions: Other Entry Dilemmas

Clair E. Martin

The exclusive right to determine who can legitimately practice within the specified activity domain of an occupation is one of the privileges granted those occupations we term professions (Freidson, 1970). In this sense, current members of a profession are the social parents of prospective replacement members, responsible for their selection and socialization to the particular knowledge, skills, and values understood to be essential for practitioners in that profession.

The requirements for entry into practice are supposed to establish the minimum qualifications necessary to protect the welfare of society and the safety and well-being of the clients served by the profession. A casual observer can readily determine that some professional groups require higher credentials for their members than do others. Closer observation reveals that the standardization of credential requirements for members is greater in some professional groups than it is in others.

This chapter will explore the entry level issues in a number of contemporary professions. As a background to these issues, a general discussion of the characteristics and processes of a profession and the related concepts of professionalism and professionalization will be presented. This foundation provides the basis for an analysis of the variation in educational level, testing, and licensing and credentialing for a selected group of professions, as well as the salient contemporary issues related to entry into practice that affect each. An underlying assumption of this paper is that variation in entry-level requirements is based primarily on the relative power wielded by the professional group. In other words, higher entry-level requirements or qualifications and a high level of standardization of members' credentials for entry into practice are a function not only of the complexity of the occupation's domain of activity but of its relative power.

WHAT IS A PROFESSION?

The concept of profession originated in the sixteenth century and referred to the university-educated occupations of divinity, law, medicine (not surgery) and "the gentlemanly occupation of the military" (Freidson, 1986, p. 22). In the same period, however, the word became associated with the full range of occupations by which people made a living. Thus, the concept was inherently ambiguous and demonstrated social ambivalence from the outset.

The broad variety of connotations associated with the term profession renders it almost useless for objective discussion. The lack of consensus on the definition and characteristics of a profession extend at least as far back as Flexner (1910). Some writers would abandon the pursuit of a definition of a profession or identification of its characteristics (Klegon, 1978; Vollmer & Mills, 1966). It is not surprising, therefore, that there should be considerable disagreement about the application of the label to specific occupations.

It is a historical fact that the term profession is a socially valued label and that there is a strong probability that both symbolic and actual social, economic, and political rewards derive from the application of that label to an occupational group. Those who have received the rewards wish to retain restricted access to them and those who have not would like to gain access to the rewards. Obviously, the concept of a profession has considerable social impact. Therefore the essential questions remain: What is a profession? How does one know whether or not professional status exists? What are the characteristics of a profession? Without conceptual clarity there is no clear guide for study or discussion related to either the process of professionalization or the structure of a profession.

Defining the Concept

There is no coherent theory of professions. The main contemporary position is to suggest construction of a theory of occupations within which professions can be treated as a special type (Freidson, 1986). Early studies of professions treated the concept generically rather than as a special type of occupation and utilized a taxonomic approach—defining the concept by listing a number of characteristics assumed always to be present. Klegon (1978) criticizes this approach as attempting a virtually impossible and unproductive task, because the concept of a profession is an ambiguous one.

One example of the taxonomic approach is the following listing of the characteristics of a professional community:

1. Its members are bound by a sense of identity.
2. Once in it, few leave, so that it is a terminal or continuing status for the most part.
3. Its members share values in common.
4. Its role definitions vis à vis both members and non-members are agreed upon and are the same for all members.
5. Within the areas of communal action there is a common language, which is understood only partially by outsiders.
6. The community has power over its members.
7. Its limits are reasonably clear, though they are not physical or geographical, but social.
8. Though it does not produce the next generation biologically, it does so socially through its control over the selection of professional trainees, and through its training processes it sends these recruits through an adult socialization process (Goode, cited in Pavalko, 1971, pp. 24–25)

Pavalko (1971) describes eight essential characteristics of professions:

1. A specific knowledge base, theory, or intellectual technique.
2. Work activities that maximize basic social values such as justice or health.
3. A fairly lengthy, specialized training period, which involves the transmission of ideational, value-laden knowledge.
4. An emphasis on service to clients and society.
5. Autonomy for both the collectivity and for individual members of the profession.

6. A strong sense of commitment to the work.

7. A community orientation in terms of shared values and norms.

8. A code of ethics.

Goode (1966) maintains that such extensive lists of traits may be subsumed under two main characteristics of a profession: "(1) prolonged specialized training in a body of abstract knowledge, and (2) a collectivity or service orientation" (p. 36). For example, he would suggest that the formulation of ethical codes is a consequence of the service orientation of the profession and its commitment to advancing the best interests of society and specific clients over the self-interest of its members.

Contemporary students of professions recognize that there is no occupation whose members all demonstrate the maximum potential of those qualities and characteristics that are associated with professional status. An additional criticism of the taxonomic approach is that an existing occupational group—generally, medicine—has served as the model for these formulations of traits (Klegon, 1978).

An alternative method of examining social phenomena is to create an ideal type—an abstraction that defines and illustrates the elements of a phenomenon, even though that exact configuration is unlikely to be found in reality. Most of the ideal-type formulations have used the same listings and characteristics as the taxonomic approach and are subject to the same criticisms. The value of establishing an ideal type, however, is that it serves as an unambiguous yardstick against which empirically observable comparisons may be made. The ideal-type approach is a significant step toward recognizing professions as a special type of occupation and not as a generic concept.

Professional Power

The concept of profession is socially defined. A profession becomes so identified by virtue of an occupational group's ability to convince society that its work is of such special value to the welfare of society and its members that the social division of labor associated with the occupation is protected and given special privileges of autonomy. The nature and powers of a profession are influenced by input from four major sources: (1) the interests of the specific occupational group, (2) legislative and governmental regulations, (3) constituent groups, and (4) the general public (Freidson, 1986).

In defining a specific profession, the occupational elite construct a reality that they hope will be accepted by the internal and external environments (Hall, 1979). The elite of a profession exercise the power to define it (Larson, 1977, pp. 226–227). The power of the elite is not independent but linked to outside power elites, including the prestige of universities, organizational clients, and connections with the state. This power is paralleled in the internal "peer esteem," excellence, and prestige or influence that the elite enjoy within the profession. To the extent that these two processes merge—that is, create a single professional hierarchy—a serious challenge from within or outside of the profession becomes less likely.

The concept of a profession is a fact of social structure. The manifest function of this social fact—the intended and recognized consequences that contribute to the adaptation of the social system—is the welfare and protection of society (Merton, 1957). The challenge of the elite is to focus the attention of the societal powers on the special knowledge and skills of the occupation that are essential to the welfare and protection of society. To ensure that the occupation is performed in such a way that the best interests of society are upheld, the profession is granted autonomy and privilege to the effect that a market monopoly is achieved—that is, competition is restricted.

Herein lies a dilemma. Is the basis for privilege the special power of the profession or the common power of vested economic, political, and bureaucratic interests (Freidson, 1986)? Whatever the basis for originally obtaining the privilege, the latent function, the unintended, unrecognized consequence, of this social fact we call a profession, is that the protected domain of activity is maintained and expanded in such a way that the self-interests of the profession are advanced. Freidson (1973) is not alone when he asserts that professional imperialism extends claims of professional knowledge and skill beyond demonstrable observations. Shimberg (1985), for example, states that while licensing is based on law and involves the police power of the state, it is nevertheless controlled by members of the profession that it is charged with regulating. A positive benefit of licensure is that a conscientious board screens and denies licenses to the unqualified. A negative consequence of licensure is that unnecessarily high standards may be applied to practitioners and unrealistically high test scores required, thereby reducing the supply of practitioners, with a consequent reduction in competition and increase in costs for services delivered. Are the careful screening, training, and credentialing of applicants into the profession a function of the concern for the welfare and protection of society or of the advancement of the status and privilege of the profession? Or are entry-into-practice requirements a combination of both latent and manifest functions that vary from one profession to another and from time to time and place to place?

This paper advances the position that the acquisition and maintenance of power and privilege are the key to an understanding of the variability of credentialing among professions and provide a basis for placing a specific occupation relative to the ideal type of profession. Freidson (1986) says that the professional associations are key to an understanding of the power of a profession insofar as the association, through legal and formal means, seeks to protect and advance the best interests of the profession. In fact, the professional elite continue to exert majority control over the boards and agencies that are constituted to provide legal control over professions and their activities.

There is a broadly held notion that the tradition of professional power and privilege is in decline as a result of a number of societal forces, including (1) the trend toward greater egalitarianism, (2) the raised level of public education, resulting in an increase in public knowledge and a decrease in professional authority, (3) consumerism, (4) the standardization and routinization of knowledge, (5) computer technology, and (6) the employment of professionals in bureaucratic settings (Freidson, 1986; Rothman, 1984). Although there is some legitimate debate concerning the impact of the social forces on established professions and their power and influence, it is safe to assume that newer and less established professions face a more resistant social climate than the laissez-faire environment that the more traditional status professions faced in their formative years.

RELATED CONCEPTS

Professionalism

The concept of a profession is a group concept and not to be confused with the individual concept of professionalism. Although individual members are expected to share certain qualities and characteristics in common, a profession is a concept of the aggregrate, a characteristic of the division of labor in the social structure. An individual is a professional by virtue of legitimate membership in a recognized profession, not as a consequence of any number of these individual qualities and characteristics. Professionalism, on the other hand, is an individual or personal attribute.

Professionalism may be a highly desirable quality for members of a profession, yet it is not directly related to professional status. One's commitment to one's career, an emphasis on service rather than profit, and conscientious ethical behavior do not establish professional status. Professional status is acquired by virtue of membership in an occupational group that has acquired the social status of a profession. When an individual says, "I am a professional," she or he is not making a statement about individual attributes, but is claiming membership in an occupation that has come to be socially recognized as a profession.

Professionalization

Professionalization is the process that the elite of a profession orchestrate as they advance the professional status of the occupation. The issue of entry into practice is one component of the social process of professionalization. Vollmer and Mills (1966) are concerned with the circumstances and processes through which an occupation becomes known as a profession. The steps in the professionalization process are: (1) higher levels of education for prospective members, (2) education by the members of the profession and not outside authorities, (3) judgment of the profession's proper work by its own members and delegation of routine matters to subordinate workers, (4) clarification of the service orientation of the occupation, and (5) research.

Goode (1966) states that "an industrializing society is a professionalizing society" (p. 902). By this he means that the complex, highly specialized division of labor characteristic of an industrial society supports and encourages the autonomous exercise of professional knowledge and skill.

The social consequences of professionalization are far-reaching. It has been a significant vehicle for individual and group social mobility; that is, enhanced social position and power in relation to others is a consequence if not a goal of professionalization.

Power is an essential resource for any occupational group seeking to transform itself into a profession (Perrucci, 1973). Larson

(1977) describes professionalization as an "attempt to translate one order of scarce resources—special knowledge and skills— into another—social and economic rewards, . . . the process by which producers of special services sought to constitute and control a market for their expertise" (p. xvii).

The historical context creates opportunities and constraints that influence the nature and characteristics of a profession (Freidson, 1986). The medieval universities gave birth to the three original professions of medicine, law, and the clergy. There was little ambiguity concerning the identity and characteristics of these professions in preindustrial Western culture. However, the onset of industrialism created a nurturing environment for the rapid growth of occupation-professions. Acquiring the status of a profession not only created the benefit of sharing the status associated with the traditional gentry, but the contemporary laissez-faire philosophy created a state-sanctioned market shelter.

Larson (1977) discusses the process by which medicine and law have acquired the unparalleled power they wield today. A summary of his discussion is provided here as an illustration of the exercise of power in controlling the marketplace and specifically in controlling the entry into practice of prospective practitioners.

The Professionalization of Medicine

During the nineteenth century the practice of medicine yielded neither higher income nor higher status than that afforded the average citizen, in spite of the physician's years of education. Specialization increased both status and income, and general practitioners looked on specialists with envy and suspicion as to their motives. Competition for clients resulted in splitting fees, and as the number of hospital beds proliferated over the turn of the century, practitioners not affiliated with hospitals or clinics raised an outcry of protest. In addition, physicians began to feel threatened by the growing numbers of trained nurses, chiropractors, and health cultists as well as by the decreased demand for their services as a result of the declining death rate due to improved health practices and antitoxins. As physicians with highly divergent interests attempted to find their own niche in the marketplace, a common concern evolved that the medical profession was overcrowded.

As these concerns began to surface, the state medical societies and the American Medical Association (AMA) became more powerful in their influence on state licensing boards and on medical schools. The more elite of the medical schools were the first to upgrade their standards and requirements; they admitted mainly students from well-to-do backgrounds who could afford to attend. It was these "elite"—better-educated specialists and scientific faculties—who became leaders in the medical societies. Meanwhile, even rural private practitioners were becoming involved in county medical societies, which became the heart of the professional association.

In 1906 all medical schools in the country were ranked by the AMA's Council on Medical Education according to a wide range of criteria, and many schools closed. A second inspection was done in 1910 by Flexner, whose report had far-reaching consequences in medical education. Flexner recommended standardization of the production of physicians and "fewer and better doctors," based on research and scientific practice. Following this report, large foundations provided some of the best and richest medical schools with more money to pursue scientific research in medicine and improve educational resources. Standards for admissions to medical schools were upgraded, and competition increased so that physicians were produced much more selectively.

Larson (1977) points out several other factors that also led to the unity of highly diverse groups and the power of organized medicine: (1) the large number of generalists and part-time specialists provided physicians with an inordinate amount of influence in shaping policies, (2) increasingly, teachers and researchers were separate from the problems of medical practice, (3) all private practitioners, general or specialists, opposed compulsory health insurance and anything else that would threaten private practice, and (4) the scarcity of new physicians ensured economic benefits to all in spite of differences among groups.

The Professionalization of Law

The profession of law is composed of even more divergent groups than is medicine. However, the strength of the American Bar Association is more the result of a careful respect for social stratification within the profession than a pulling together of diverse groups around a common interest. The major factor that established law as a powerful and influential profession was the need of businesses for legal advice and counsel. At the end of the last century, railroad general counsel, corporate counsel, and counsel for investment bankers made a place for lawyers in the upper echelons of business management in America.

At the same time there was a move to upgrade the profession, requiring graduation from law school rather than apprenticeship training. Law schools became active participants in the professionalization of law and the standardization of requirements for the bar. In spite of the standardization of training, the profession is highly stratified, with prestigious law schools producing lawyers who join prestigious law firms or corporations, serving prestigious clients, and careful segregation of different areas of practice. At every level, members of the bar have in common a dependence on the "stability and legitimacy of a given institutional and legal framework" (Larson, 1977, p. 168), as well as the clients whom they serve. Economic and professional status thus rely on the careful nurture of both clients and the existing system of justice.

ENTRY-INTO-PRACTICE REQUIREMENTS AND ISSUES

The remainder of this chapter analyzes the variability of requirements for entry into practice both among and within a number of selected professions. The majority of the professions that are regulated by the state are health-related occupations, as reflected in the number of such professions discussed here. Most of the information which follows was taken from the 1986–87 edition of the *Occupational Outlook Handbook* (Bureau of Labor Statistics, 1986). Confirmation of this material and discussion of issues came from personal communication with members of the respective professional associations.

Table 1 summarizes the educational, experience, licensing, and credentialing requirements for entry into practice and identifies major contemporary issues for these selected professions. A more detailed discussion of each profession follows.

Architecture

Architects must be registered or licensed in all 50 states in order to provide architectural services, and a registered architect is required to be legally responsible for all work. In order to qualify for the examination the applicant must have a minimum of a bachelor of architecture (a five-year degree) and three years' experience in the field (working for a registered architect). The de-

TABLE 1
Requirements for Entry into Selected Professions

Profession	Degree Level for Entry	Testing	License or Certificate	Current Issues
Architecture	BA	Exam and experience	X	Nature of required work experience
Clergy	Varies greatly	None required	Ordination	
Dentistry	DDS/ DMD	Written and practical	X	State reciprocity for licensing
Education	BS	17 states	X	Competency exam; raising educational level
Engineering	BS	Exam and experience	*	
Law	JD or LLB	Exam	X	Timing of bar exam
Medicine	MD/DO	Exam and experience	X	
Nursing	Diploma/ ADN/ BSN/ MN	Exam	X	Raising educational level
Occupational therapy	BS or MS	29 states	36 states	Raising educational level
Optometry	DO	Exam	X	
Pharmacy	BS/ PharmD	Exam and experience	X	One degree
Physical therapy	BS/MS	Exam	X	Raising educational level
Social work	BSW/BA		33 states	Licensure
Speech pathology	MS	Exam and experience	36 states	Licensure
Veterinary medicine	DVM/ VMD	Exam	X	Standard exam

*Those whose work may affect life, health, or property, or who offer public service.

gree must come from one of 92 schools accredited by the National Architectural Accrediting Board. The examination is a standardized one from the National Council of Architectural Registration Examining Boards (B. Kimberlin, American Institute of Architects, personal communication, September 15, 1986).

Clergy

The clergy were once regarded as a prestigious profession, particularly before the Reformation, when they were the representatives of the powerful Roman Catholic Church. Contemporary clergymen and women do not wield much power as a profession. Although many religions require a bachelor's degree and a number of years of seminary for ordination, others have no educational qualifications for those members receiving a "call" to serve. There are no state regulations concerning qualifications for clergymen or women. Ordination by a recognized church or religion is valid for performance of marriage ceremonies.

Dentistry

Dentists must be licensed in all 50 states. Qualifications include graduation with a DDS or DMD from a dental school approved by the Commission on Dental Accreditation and successful completion of both a written and practical exam. In nearly all states, the written exam is one given by the National Board of Dental Examiners. The major entry issue facing the dental profession in this country is state reciprocity for licensing. Many states require that a practical exam be passed even by a dentist who is licensed and has been practicing in another state (R. Weathers, Dean, College of Dentistry, Emory University, personal communication, August 1986).

Education

Public school teachers in all states are required to have a teaching certificate, which can be obtained if one has a bachelor's degree, including specific required courses in the teacher's subject area and in education, as well as student teaching experience. At least 17 states now require applicants for certification to pass a competency test in basic skills, subject matter, teaching skills, or a combination of these. Health requirements must also be met in 20 states. Teachers are expected to continue their education in order to continue to be certified in most states. Validation of teachers' competency and increasing the level of education are the major entry issues in education.

Engineering

Engineers may be involved in many specialties and the requirements for each specialty differ. However, those engineers "whose work may affect life, health, or property, or who offer services to the public" (Bureau of Labor Statistics, 1986, p. 62) must be licensed in all 50 states. In most states a license requires that the applicant be a graduate of an accredited program in engineering and have four years of engineering experience prior to writing an eight-hour exam, which is uniform for all states. The engineer is then registered as a Professional Engineer. Further certification in a specialty may be required. The National Council of Engineering Examiners has set up a model law as a goal for state licensure laws (Jean Robertson, National Society of Professional Engineers, personal communication, September 16, 1986).

Law

Lawyers must be admitted to the bar in the state in which they wish to practice, following successful completion of a bar examination. The applicant must have completed at least three years of college and graduated from a law school approved by the American Bar Association. At least one state, Georgia, allows students to write the bar exam in the last semester of law school. The degree earned is either a JD or LLB. Most states require the exam to be taken for admission to that state bar, although there is some state reciprocity, provided certain conditions are met. Many states use the Multistate Bar Examination as a part of the state bar exam, in addition to an ethics examination (D. Epstein, Dean, Law School, Emory University, personal communication, August 1986).

Medicine

Physicians also have strict requirements for entry into the profession. Applicants must have completed medical school in an accredited institution and have had one or two years of supervised practice (internship/residency) in an accredited graduate program before writing the exam for licensure. The National Board of Medical Examiners examination is accepted by all states except Texas and Louisiana.

Nursing

Nurses must be registered following successful completion of the National Council Licensure Examination (NCLEX) administered by each state. The exam may be taken following completion of several different levels of education: a three-year diploma program, a two-year associate degree program, a four-year bachelor's degree program, or in a few cases, a generic master's degree program. Nursing is currently attempting to resolve this problem of the wide variation in entry-level requirements and upgrade the minimum credential for entry into practice to the bachelor's degree, a controversial issue.

Occupational Therapy

Thirty-six states require a license for occupational therapists. Qualifications for licensure include graduation from an accredited program and certification by a standardized examination from the American Occupational Therapy Association. Occupational therapists enter the profession at one of three educational levels: (1) with a bachelor's degree in occupational therapy, (2) with a post-baccalaureate certificate, earned by persons with a bachelor's degree in another field, usually requiring about two years of further schooling, or (3) with a professional master's degree, also available for those who have a baccalaureate degree in another area. Occupational therapists are attempting to get licensure in every state. They are also considering a graduate degree as a minimum for entry into practice; this concern has more to do with the content of the education than with the type of degree. The amount of work required to obtain the bachelor's degree is assumed to normally qualify a person for a graduate degree (S. Hoover, American

Occupational Therapy Association, personal communication, September 15, 1986).

Optometry

Optometrists must have a doctor of optometry degree from an accredited program and pass a state board examination to be licensed in all states. There is some reciprocity between states.

Pharmacy

Pharmacists are quite strictly controlled. In all states, licensure requires graduation from an accredited pharmacy program, successful completion of a state board examination (standardized in all but three states), a specified amount of practical experience, and demonstration of good character. The PharmD (six years) and the BPharm (five years) degrees are both entry-level degrees for pharmacists. The PharmD degree may also be earned by licensed pharmacists at a higher level, although it is not treated as a graduate degree. Pharmacists are aggressively recruited by potential employers and are in short supply. Members of the profession would like to see only one degree offered, but there is continuing debate as to which it would be. Potential employers are concerned that a shortfall of graduates would occur if all programs were to switch to the six-year PharmD degree; educators are concerned about a need for extra resources and perhaps decreased class size; professionals are questioning the use of the term "doctor" when so many members of the profession are educated at the baccalaureate level. A number of experimental, nontraditional programs are seeking to offer the PharmD degree to licensed pharmacists with the BPharm, in an attempt to explore the possibility of upgrading educational levels of experienced pharmacists (R. Penna, American Association of Colleges of Pharmacy, personal communication, September 16, 1986).

Physical Therapy

Physical therapists also have several entry levels: a bachelor's degree in physical therapy, a certificate from programs for students who already have a bachelor's degree in another field, or a master's degree in physical therapy. A license is required in all states. Applicants must have one of the listed degrees and write an examination, which is uniform in all states, to be licensed. The profession is currently attempting to raise entry-level requirements to the master's degree level by 1990 (K. Davis, American Physical Therapy Association, personal communication, September 15, 1986).

Social Work

Social workers recognize three levels of education: (1) the bachelor of social work degree, (2) the master's in social work, and (3) the independent level, which involves several years of higher education and practice. Thirty-nine states have laws regarding licensing or registration of social workers. These laws vary but include holding a minimum of a BSW and writing an exam which is uniform for all states but two. Social workers may be voluntarily certified by the National Association of Social Workers (NASW). Myles Johnson (personal communication, September 15, 1986) of NASW points out several disturbing trends. First, a large number of people who are not trained in social work are filling social work positions. This goes along with a trend among both public and private employers toward "declassification"—removing the requirement for a social work degree in order to save money. Finally, there is little recognition of the difference between the levels of education in terms of job responsibilities. Social workers in state chapters of NASW are pushing for stronger state licensure.

Speech Pathology

Speech-language pathology and audiology is licensed in 36 states, with audiology licensed in one additional state. Applicants must have a master's degree in speech-language pathology or audiology and 300 hours' supervised clinical experience to write the examination. The exam is uniform for all states. The American Speech-Language-Hearing Association (ASHA) is a certifying agent, requiring the same qualifications as the license; therefore, a certificate from ASHA is sufficient for licensure in all 36 states. The association is working for licensure in all states. Certification may eventually require a PhD, but not in the near future (D. Cahill, American Speech-Language-Hearing Association, personal communication, September 15, 1986).

Veterinary Medicine

Veterinarians must be licensed to practice in all states. Licensure requires a DVM or VMD from an accredited veterinary medicine program, and successful completion of a written National Board Exam. Twenty-six states require the written Clinical Competency Test; the others use some combination of oral and practical examination, which may not be legally defensible. Licensing procedures in some states may be influenced by the perception of an oversupply of veterinarians. A major research project is now underway to use criterion-referenced testing for the National Boards, which are currently norm-based (E. R. Ames, American Veterinary Medical Association, personal communication, September 15, 1986).

CONCLUSION

This review illustrates the dynamic state of entry-level requirements, not only for the younger, less secure professions, but for the older "status" professions as well. There is an obvious tension between the "deprofessionalization" social forces that seek to limit the power of the professions and the efforts of the professions themselves to increase their relative status through an increase in the qualifications and credentials of their members and to control the marketplace through use of the service ideal rationale.

The greatest variability in the level of education required for entry into practice is found among those professions that have relatively less social power and whose members include a majority of women and are primarily employed in institutions and agencies. These professions also tend to be obligated to implement delegated functions from other professions in the course of meeting their employment responsibilities.

The variation in testing for entry into practice does not follow this pattern. Rather, variability in theoretical and practical examination tends to be greater among those professions that have relatively greater power and that have economic incentives to reduce competition in the marketplace.

Entry-into-practice issues are one component of the overall professionalization process pursued by professional occupations. As such, they are subject to historical social forces that vary from time to time as well as geographically. Attempting to understand these issues in isolation from the historical social context may lead to an incomplete and misleading understanding. This chapter has suggested that it is the relative power of an occupation that enables it to standardize the requirements for entry into practice that have been determined to be in the best interests of the profession by its elite. The exercise of power is always implemented in a specific historical and social context and it is this context that either enhances or restrains the acquisition and exercise of power.

REFERENCES

Bureau of Labor Statistics. (1986). *Occupational Outlook Handbook, 1986–87*. Washington, DC: U.S. Department of Labor.

Cullen, J. B. (1985). Professional differentiation and occupational earnings. *Work & Occupations, 12*, 351–372.

Dingwall, R., & Lewis, P. (Eds.). (1983). *The sociology of the professions: Lawyers, doctors and others*. New York: St. Martin's.

Flexner, A. (1910). *Medical education in the United States and Canada: A report to the Carnegie Foundation for the advancement of teaching*. New York: Carnegie Foundation.

Forsyth, P. B., & Danisiewiz, T. J. (1985). Toward a theory of professionalism. *Work & Occupations, 12*, 59–76.

Freidson, E. (1970). *Profession of medicine: A study of the sociology of applied knowledge*. New York: Dodd, Mead.

Freidson, E. (Ed.). (1973). *The professions and the prospects*. Beverly Hills, CA: Sage.

Freidson, E. (1986). *Professional powers: A study of the institutionalization of formal knowledge*. Chicago: University of Chicago.

Geison, G. L. (Ed.). (1983). *Professions and professional ideologies in America*. Chapel Hill: University of North Carolina.

Goode, W. (1966). "Professions" and "non-professions." In H. M. Vollmer & D. L. Mills (Eds.), *Professionalization*. Englewood Cliffs, NJ: Prentice-Hall.

Hall, R. (1979). The social construction of the professions. *Sociology of Work and Occupations, 6*, 124–126.

Johnson, T. J. (1972). *Professions and power*. London: Macmillan.

Klegon, D. (1978). The sociology of professions: An emerging perspective. *Sociology of Work and Occupations, 5*, 259–283.

Larson, M. S. (1977). *The rise of professionalism: A sociological analysis*. Berkeley, CA: University of California.

Merton, R. K. (1957). *Social theory and social structure*. New York: Free Press.

Otto, L. B., Call, V. R. A., & Spenner, K. I. (1981). *Design for a study of entry*. Lexington, MA: D. C. Heath.

Pavalko, R. M. (1971). *Sociology of occupations and professions*. Itasca, IL: F. E. Peacock.

Perrucci, R. (1973). Engineering: Professional servant of power. In E. Freidson (Ed.), *The professions and their prospects*. Beverly Hills, CA: Sage.

Rothman, R. A. (1984). Deprofessionalization: The case of law in America. *Work and Occupations, 11*, 183–206.

Shimberg, B. (1985). Overview of professional and occupational licensing. In J. C. Fortune & Associates (Eds.). *Understanding testing in occupational licensing*. San Francisco: Jossey-Bass.

Vollmer, H. M., & Mills, D. L. (Eds.). (1966). *Professionalization*. Englewood Cliffs, NJ: Prentice-Hall.

PART II

Educational Issues

CHAPTER 3

Competencies of Associate and Professional Nurses

Vivien DeBack

Throughout the recent history of nursing, there have been a number of trends and fads that began slowly, and then spread across the profession. Ultimately, each idea was either adopted as a standard for the profession or dropped as unusable or unacceptable. Competence statements describing the abilities of the graduates of associate degree and bachelor's degree nursing programs may be just such a trend. They have developed slowly over time and have increased in both number and type.

In this instance, however, the development of competence statements has not followed the usual pattern. Rather than either rejecting or accepting them, nursing seems to be fixated at the development or refinement stage of competence statements and unable to determine their best use.

The competence statements referred to here are descriptions of nurses' behaviors (cognitive, affective, and psychomotor) that are amenable to assessment and that differentiate two categories of nursing practice. These statements have been developed by nurse educators, practitioners, and administrators to describe the abilities of the new graduate. They are considered to describe the outcomes of the educational program as well as the abilities of the beginning practitioner.

NCNIP'S ANALYSIS OF COMPETENCE STATEMENTS

The staff of the National Commission on Nursing Implemation Project (NCNIP) became involved in the content analysis of competence statements when the project's Work Group on Education needed such information for their deliberations. This work group was responsible for reviewing existing data on the establishment of two categories of nurses and determining the level of consensus in the nursing community on this issue. The statements collected represented a range of national, regional, state, and local groups, and the review indicated that they were developed to define the competencies that characterize nurses prepared in associate degree nursing (ADN) and baccalaureate degree nursing (BSN) programs (National Commission on Nursing Implementation Project, 1985).

All competence statements reviewed by the NCNIP staff were developed by groups of nursing educators, practitioners, and administrators who were elected or appointed to committees or task forces responsible for this activity. (A list of the statements reviewed is appended to this chapter.) Many of the documents refer to major nursing studies that have recommended the creation of two categories of nursing practice as the motivation for their work in developing competence statements.

Preliminary comments made in these documents indicate that the basis for the competence statements was a belief that the role of nurse encompasses differentiated levels of functions, which result in collaborative, interdependent, and complementary parameters of practice. These functions are believed to be consistent with the educational preparation of a specific practitioner. It is interesting to note that the groups that gave specific guidelines about what was meant by the notion of a competence did not seem to produce a significantly different document from groups that did not define the concept at all. Most documents suggest that the two new categories of nurse should share a core of knowledge and skills but at the same time remain distinct in terms of accountability and depth and breadth of practice. Most statements suggest that ADN and BSN competencies will be used to guide curriculum development as well as patterns of utilization for nurses in the practice setting.

Based on their content analysis of the competence statements, the NCNIP staff classified the statements into three major categories:

- Identification of competencies about which there is consistent agreement in the data, which either describe commonalities in ADN and BSN practice (consensus) or differentiate between ADN and BSN practice (consensus).
- Identification of inconsistency in the data (consensus not achieved).
- Identification of competencies that are unique to one kind of preparation and regarding which there is no corresponding competence statement for the other category of practice.

Very few statements were classified as "consensus not achieved." Where consensus was achieved, a fairly clear picture of differentiated practice began to emerge. The major differences between ADN and BSN practice noted in the statements focused on the type of client (patient condition) and the environment for practice (structure and support). Thus, the associate degree nurse cares for clients with common, well-defined nursing diagnoses in structured health care settings with established policies, procedures, and protocols. The BSN cares for clients with complex interactions of nursing diagnoses in both structured and unstructured settings, which have the potential for variations requiring independent nursing decisions.

The proliferation of competence statements since the mid-1970s and the commonalities noted among statements developed by such diverse groups as the American Nurses' Association, the National League for Nursing's Council of Associate Degree Programs, the Wisconsin Task Force, and so forth, seem to suggest a wide acceptance of differentiated practice and differentiated educational outcomes between ADN and BSN nurses. However, the development and dissemination of these statements has not resolved the issue of differentiated practice for graduates of associate degree and BSN programs; and, as noted earlier, the nursing community cannot seem to move beyond this developmental stage to implementation. Two major issues seem to relate to this fixation: (1) the nature of the expectations regarding the problem that competence statements were meant to solve and (2) the "present" rather than "future" orientation of the statements.

EXPECTATIONS FOR COMPETENCE STATEMENTS

Competence statements were intended to solve a practice problem, but they were developed as if they were addressing an educational problem. The expectation was that if educators defined the products of their programs quite clearly, it would solve the problem of differentiating the functions of the two categories of nurses in practice. Competencies seem to reflect quite clearly the outcomes of education as defined by associate and baccalaureate program educators. In addition, they seem to differentiate two categories of beginning practice for graduates of ADN and BSN programs. Why then have these rather widely accepted statements of differentiation not been effective in resolving the two category dilemma in practice?

The literature related to competence statements does not help to answer that question. Many articles and research projects related to competencies focus on the perceptions of faculty or nursing service personnel regarding ADN or BSN graduates' performance in the specified areas (Chamings & Teevan, 1979; Hayter, 1971); graduates' perceptions of their own performance (Nelson, 1978) or educational preparedness (Hogstel, 1977); or the extent to which graduates demonstrate a specific behavior or behaviors (Matthews & Gaul, 1979). Chamings and Teevan (1979) concluded that "current evidence is inadequate to tell whether graduates of different types of programs actually perform differently" (p. 18). Indeed, collecting evidence on differentiated performance in settings that do not provide for such differentation may have slowed the process of applying the competencies as a basis for the practice roles of associate- and baccalaureate-prepared nurses in service.

It is true that common licensure for both ADN and BSN graduates is often considered the culprit blocking differentiated practice. A more likely cause, however, is the practice arena, which neither supports nor rewards nurses who perform as their educational outcomes indicate they can or should practice.

Only recently have competence statements defining differentiated educational outcomes been made the basis for development of differentiated job descriptions and been tested in the clinical setting (Primm, 1986). Data are now being collected on the effectiveness and efficiency of differentiated practice in hospital settings (Rotkovitch, 1986). This step, taken more then ten years after competence statements began to proliferate, is not widely accepted. However, the use of competencies to develop job descriptions and to provide direction for the organization of the clinical environment seem to be a most appropriate application for these documents. Without a national plan to develop appropriate clinical utilization of different practitioners, there is little likelihood that competence statements will serve as a basis for differentiation in practice.

It is important to note that competence statements do not define the totality of the domain of nursing. The integration of cognitive, affective, and psychomotor skills is an intellectual process not easily defined by independent, discrete abilities. Competence statements are not descriptive of the full scope of nursing practice. Competence statements do not resolve licensure issues, except to ensure that different categories of practice are indeed different and therefore amenable to differentiated licenses. Competence statements do not resolve the titling issue, except to point out that differentiated practice suggests different titles for the consumer's benefit.

Competence statements are helpful in giving direction to educators in preparing graduates. They are helpful to nursing service in the development of job descriptions and in organizing the milieu for nursing practice.

The development of competence statements as a solution to an educational problem rather than as a solution to a practice dilemma may well result in their rejection by the profession as a passing fad rather than an enduring and ultimately accepted trend.

"PRESENT" ORIENTATION OF COMPETENCE STATEMENTS

A second issue related to use of the competence statements is their orientation to the present rather than the future of nursing practice. Competencies generally describe the outcomes of educational programs at the time that the statements were written. Although it may be true that competence statements were believed to be a road map to the future by assisting the profession to tie educational preparation to the service milieu, it is also true that the statements themselves do not describe future practice. They have been developed by faculty and practitioners who described the service needs and educational preparation in the current system.

Just as the competence statements that have been around for eight to ten years have not helped us to solve the practice problem of differentiating competencies in practice, those same competence statements will not be effective road maps to the future if they are used as final, static products. The statements could be helpful to the nursing community if they are seen as part of a process of change, as useful conduits to the future, while nursing practice and practice settings continue to evolve.

The statements have been developed for a health care system that no longer exists. The current system is in a state of flux. The existing competence statements may not be helpful for either practice or education in a future, structurally different system that is highly competitive, multitiered, and technologically advanced. Therefore, we must consider the statements themselves to be in flux and expect them to be refined and revised as the system and the profession changes. It appears that another expectation—that the competence statements would help lead us to the future— and the basis for development in present practice and knowledge may have helped to fixate the competence statements at the development level.

WHERE DO WE GO FROM HERE?

The competencies that have been developed must be moved from the educational to the practice arena. Given the assumption that nursing educators agree that the ADN and BSN competencies do in fact describe their graduates, the next step is the redesign of the practice settings to support, encourage, reward, and expect differentiated practice based in these competencies.

Perhaps this change has yet to take place because nursing service in organized settings does not see the value of differentiated practice. However, we have yet to demonstrate that the use of competence statements as the basis for differentiated job descriptions contributes to high-quality, cost-effective nursing service. A few service institutions are in the process of piloting differentiated job descriptions that will provide this much-needed data (Primm, 1986).

If nursing is to move into differentiated practice, all nursing service administrators will need baseline data to compare with information gathered once differentiated practice is introduced into their setting. These data must include current nursing service costs and data on the level of care currently being delivered. The need to gather such information places a substantial burden on nursing administrators in acute-care, long-term care, and home care agencies. The following are the steps that must be considered in preparing this data:

1. *Delineate levels of practice based on a needs assessment of the clients the agency serves.* The nursing administrator must identify the needs of the population in the agency to de-

termine the type of practitioners to assign to each unit. Many agencies will find that tools they already are using for patient classification will assist them with this assessment. Some areas of the agency will need an all-BSN staff. Others may require a BSN coordinator with several ADN staff, while others may need a still different mix.

2. *Use present cost data to project future costs based on nursing care needs.* If the agency does not have current data on the cost of nursing care, a cost accounting must be done so that this baseline data can be used for future forecasting and comparison. Assuming that such costs are available and a needs assessment has been made, projection of future costs can be determined. Some units of the agency will probably be more costly than others; however, those costs can be justified with data from the needs assessment. Various nurse staffing mixes can be assigned to different areas to collect data on their effectiveness and efficiency.

3. *Develop job descriptions of differentiated practice based on ADN and BSN competencies.* Although each agency has some unique features, existing job descriptions can be used as a starting point to begin to define differentiated practice (Primm, 1986; Rotkovitch, 1986). Many agencies have job descriptions related to clinical career ladders that might serve as the basis for ADN and BSN practice in their institution.

4. *Reorganize the nursing delivery system, assigning appropriate categories of nurses to each unit or section of the agency.* A trial period in one unit for testing differentiated job descriptions may be helpful in introducing the new concept of practice into an agency. As with most change, allowing time for development and staff input is critical to the success of implementation. The speed with which change occurs depends on the effectiveness of the plan developed for implementation, the mix of nurses already in the agency, the clarity of the job descriptions, and success in convincing every nurse that her or his services are valued.

5. *Collect data on effectiveness and efficiency of units or sections of the agency.* A decision about data collection should be made prior to implementing differentiated practice. The administrator should begin by assessing the types of data that already exist that might be useful in determining the effectiveness and efficiency of the unit. Patient data such as

length of stay, recidivism rate, infections and incidents, and satisfaction with care are useful. Determine what other data are needed, who will collect and analyze it, and who will report the findings.

6. *Compare new data on cost and quality to data collected under the former system.* A period of time after start-up is needed before data collected can be considered valid. A good plan could be implemented in six months, and data could be collected soon after.

These steps are necessary if nursing is going to move the competence statements of differentiated education into the practice arena. In their needs assessment, some nursing administrators may find a need for numbers of associate degree nurses, with baccalaureate nurses in leadership positions, while others may find a need for all baccalaureate nurses. In this changing health care environment, both baccalaureate and associate degree nurses are valued and needed.

CONCLUSION

It has been suggested here that the fixation of competence statements for ADN and BSN nursing practice at the development level is due to expectations of the type of problem that the statements were meant to solve, and to the orientation of the competencies described to current rather than future nursing practice. Both issues can be dealt with if and when the practice setting values and makes provisions for differentiated practice. To ignore this responsibility is to invite continued confusion on practice issues involving ADN and BSN nurses.

COMPETENCE STATEMENTS REVIEWED BY NCNIP

American Nurses' Association. (1981). *Educational preparation for nursing. A source book.* Kansas City, MO: American Nurses' Association.

Midwest Alliance in Nursing. (1985). *Associate Degree Nursing: Facilitating competency development, defining and differentiating nursing competencies.* Unpublished report.

National League for Nursing, Council of Associate Degree Programs. (1978). *Competencies of the associate degree nurse on entry into practice.* New York: National League for Nursing.

National League for Nursing, Council of Baccalaureate and Higher Degree Programs. (1979). *Characteristics of baccalaureate education in nursing*. New York: National League for Nursing.

New York State Nurses' Association, Council of Nursing Education. (1978). *Report of the task force on behavioral outcomes of nursing education programs*. Unpublished report.

North Dakota Board of Nursing. (In press). *Administrative rules, article 54-03.1, requirements for nursing education program*. Submitted to the North Dakota Legislative Council for publication in the Administrative Code Supplement.

Texas Nurses' Association, Council on Education. (1983). *Directions for nursing education in Texas 1983–1995: An operational plan*. Unpublished report.

Vermont Nurses' Association. (1985). *Vermont Registered Nurse, 51*(4).

Wisconsin Task Force. (1982). *Competencies of two levels of nurses*. Madison: Wisconsin Task Force.

REFERENCES

Chamings, P., & Teevan, J. (1979, February). Comparison of expected competencies of baccalaureate and associate degree graduates in nursing. *Image, 11*(1), 16–21.

Hayter, M. (1971). Follow-up study of graduates of the University of Kentucky, College of Nursing, 1964–1969. *Nursing Research, 20*, 55–60.

Hogstel, M. (1977). Associate degree and baccalaureate graduates: Do they function differently? *American Journal of Nursing, 77*, 1598–1600.

Matthews, C., & Gaul, A. L. (1979). Nursing diagnosis from the perspectives of concept attainment and critical thinking. *Advances in Nursing Science, 2*, 17–26.

National Commission on Nursing Implementation Project (1985). *Content analysis of associate degree and baccalaureate degree competencies*. Unpublished paper, National Commission on Nursing Implementation Project, Milwaukee, WI.

Nelson, L. (1978, March–April). Competencies of nursing graduates in technical, communicative and administrative skills. *Nursing Research, 27*(2) 121–125.

Primm, P. (1986, May–June). Entry into practice: Competency statements for BSN's and ADN's. *Nursing Outlook*, 135–137.

Rotkovitch, R. (1986, June). ICON: A model of nursing practice for the future. *Nursing Management, 17*(6), 54–56.

CHAPTER 4

Mobility Programs for Students and Faculty

Sylvia E. Hart and Theresa G. Sharp

CAREER MOBILITY FOR STUDENTS

A few decades ago, hospital-based diploma programs began to give way to academic nursing programs. Associate degree nursing programs were initiated at a prolific rate, and baccalaureate programs became commonplace on college and university campuses. It appeared that an intelligent and understandable system for the delivery of nursing education would become a reality. It soon became apparent, however, that the development of the system was hampered by a series of ponderous licensure and practice questions, as well as by questions raised both by proponents of the "separate and distinct" concept of nursing careers and by those who viewed nursing as one career with multiple options for lateral and upward development. Some of these questions have now been answered. Others are still being debated. But it is clear that many practical nurses and associate degree and diploma-prepared registered nurses are finding ways to upgrade their academic credentials and, in that process, are "climbing the career ladder."

The career ladder concept is a way of visualizing an individual moving upward within a career, with each rung representing a higher academic degree or credential. For the nursing career ladder, the bottom rung is conceptualized as the certificate conferred upon completion of an LPN program. The second rung is the associate degree, the third rung is the baccalaureate, the fourth rung is the MSN degree, and the fifth rung is the nursing doctorate.

There are at least two problems with the ladder analogy. The first is that most people who climb a ladder begin at the bottom rung, whereas in nursing people can enter the system on any one of the rungs. The second is that the proper placement of the diploma rung is shrouded in ambiguity, despite the fact that thousands of registered nurses have entered the career system at that level.

The Terminology of Career Mobility

Perhaps because the career ladder analogy falls short of completely describing the way people enter and move through the nursing education system, or perhaps because the system itself is so multifaceted, the number of terms currently utilized to describe the phenomenon of career mobility is almost infinite. Some of the terms are useful and appear to be well understood by those most affected by them. Others appear to serve no useful purpose or, even worse, add confusion and ambiguity to a situation that begs for clarity and specificity. Consider for a moment that the literature on the subject of career mobility uses, with varying degrees of consistency, such terms as "open door" (Waters, 1976), "open learning" (Lenburg, 1975), "open curriculum" (Walsh, 1975; Sorensen, 1976), "open admission" (Lenburg, 1975), "career mobility" (Smailer, 1979), "career ladder" (Bullough, 1979; Sorensen, 1976), "multiple entry" (Notter & Robey, 1979), "multiple exit" (Directory of Career Mobility Programs, 1976; Sorensen, 1976), "articulation programs" (Hall, 1979; Sorensen, 1976; Stevens, 1981; Zusey, 1986), "two-plus-two programs" (Galliford, 1980), and "generic programs" (Bullough, 1979; Gross & Bevil, 1981).

Another list of terms is used to describe the methodology for facilitating or achieving career mobility. These terms include, but are not limited to, "challenge examination" (Hale & Boyd, 1981; Sorensen, 1976), "credit-by-examination" (Burnside, 1969; Hangartner, 1966; MacLean, Knoll, & Kinney, 1985), "independent study" (Walsh, 1975), "advanced placement" (MacLean, Knoll, & Kinney, 1985; Malkin, 1966), and "professional portfolio" (Marsh & Lasky, 1984). A third group of terms is used to describe the mode of program delivery. "Accelerated program" (Kramer, 1970; Laverdier, 1973), "external degree program" (Wozniak, 1973), "consortium" (Bullough, 1979), "weekend college" (Davis, Shiber, & Allen, 1984), "flexible process" (Reed, 1979), and "advanced competency program and externship" (Allison, Balmat, Keheley, Shoptaw, Anderson, Hinton, & King, 1984), are examples of terms used to describe how programs are delivered.

If we can accept as one simple definition of career mobility that it is a process of career advancement through additional education, some of these terms become redundant. Other terms such as open curriculum, articulation, validation of prior learning, and flexibility, which appear to be most often associated with career mobility, are more critical to our understanding of the notion. These four terms recur whether the reference is to LPNs moving into ADN programs (Drage, 1971; Fasano, 1976; Lenburg & Rapaport, 1979; Moore, 1981) or to RNs moving into BSN programs (Boyle, 1972; Bullough, 1972; Lenburg & Johnson, 1974; Stevens, 1981; Styles & Wilson, 1979; Zusey, 1986).

The term "open curriculum" evolved when it became apparent that not every nursing student needed to begin at the beginning of a nursing program, that the content of nursing programs of various types was not mutually exclusive, and that nursing students, like the population at large, acquire knowledge and develop skills in a variety of ways. Notter and Robey (1979) note that some time in the 1960s, nurse educators began to realize that in the process of passing the licensure examination, RNs had already demonstrated nursing knowledge that should not be ignored when determining placement in a baccalaureate nursing program. A definition of the open curriculum put forward by Waters ten years ago seems to be congruent with current thinking on the subject. Waters (1976) wrote that the

open curriculum in nursing education is a system which takes into account the different purposes of the various types of programs but recognizes common areas of achievement. Such a system permits student mobility in light of their ability, changing career goals, and changing aspirations. It also requires clear delineation of the achievement expectations of nursing programs from practical nursing through graduate education. It recognizes the possibility of mobility from other health-related fields. It is an interrelated system of achievement in nursing education with "open doors," rather than quantitative serial steps [p. 3].

The term "articulation" is also in common use. Webster's defines *articulation* as "the way in which parts are joined together" and indicates that to articulate is "to arrange in connected sequence; to fit together." There are wide variations, however, in how well nursing programs do articulate with one another and less than total agreement about whether or how completely they *should* articulate with one another. The fact is that if the nursing education system was perfectly articulated, there would be no need to validate prior knowledge or even to have an open curriculum. The LPN curriculum would constitute the first year of the associate degree curriculum, the associate degree curriculum would constitute the first two years of the BSN curriculum, the BSN curriculum would constitute the essential prerequisite for the MSN curriculum, and the MSN curriculum would be an integral component of the doctoral nursing program. Because this is clearly not the case in the real world of nursing education, nurse educators in all types of nursing programs throughout the country have felt compelled to validate, measure, assess, or otherwise determine exactly what each applicant knows and can do, unless the applicant is willing to "begin at the beginning" of the program.

Approaches to this problem have varied from the now nearly defunct blanket credit approach to an elaborate series of testing and demonstration activities. The blanket credit approach was commonplace in the 1950s and early 1960s, was used almost exclusively to award academic credit for diploma nursing courses, and was based on the assumption that licensed graduates of diploma programs had learned something about nursing. The sophisticated theoretical and clinical testing programs currently in use are based on the assumption that absolutely nothing can be taken for granted about what anyone knows about anything. As is usually the case, the truth of the matter may lie midway between these approaches, but it is clear that attempts are now being made to establish a strong and logical relationship between the awarding of academic credit and what the student has mastered.

The term "flexibility" utilized within the context of career mobility sometimes refers to the mechanisms used to determine advanced placement or to award academic credit, but more often refers to the convenience and accessibility of the program. Several models for program delivery have emerged. At one extreme is the more traditional model in which, although some courses may be passed by challenge examinations, the remainder of the courses must be taken on a college or university campus with other students as part of a full-time day program. At the other extreme is a program that can be completed without enrolling in any courses at all. Between these two extremes are such approaches as the weekend college; self-paced, modularized, independent study courses; or a combination of traditional course work with individualized clinical learning experiences.

There are those who contend that too much flexibility results in a loss of quality control. Others believe that too little flexibility is counterproductive to the concept of career mobility. In this regard it is useful to recall that, as early as 1970, the Board of Directors of the National League for Nursing went on record in support of the open curriculum. The board's statement expressed the belief that individuals who wished to change their career goals should be able to do so, but added the cautionary note that "upward mobility opportunities should be provided without lowering standards" (National League for Nursing, 1970). In other words, no teaching or program methods are automatically off limits, as long as the accepted standards for higher education are maintained.

Maintaining Standards

Given this position, it is imperative that, as nurse educators become more facilitative in providing career mobility opportunities for students from a variety of backgrounds, they keep before them the quality standards inherent in associate degree and baccalaureate education. Above all else, nursing degrees at these two levels must have the same credibility and garner the same respect as those same degrees have when they are earned in other disciplines or are acquired in more traditional nursing programs. To that end, it is useful to review the history and meaning of these two academic degrees.

The first associate degrees in the United States were awarded in 1900 by the University of Chicago after students completed the first two years of an undergraduate program. Since that time, associate degrees have been conferred by some four-year colleges and universities, but the vast majority of these degrees are now conferred by junior and community colleges (Spurr, 1970). The point is that the associate degree is conferred when students successfully complete the equivalent of what most people view as the first half of a baccalaureate program.

Baccalaureate programs typically require the equivalent of four years of full-time study, and, in addition to many of the same course requirements that characterize associate degree programs,

include a broader range of general or liberal education requirements and in-depth exploration of a major field of study at the
upper-division level (*Integrity in the College Curriculum*, 1985).

To maintain the meaning and integrity of these two degrees, it
is incumbent on nurse educators who are facilitating career mobility for students to award college credit only for college-level
work. More specifically, they must award lower-division credit
for lower-division work and upper-division credit only for upper-
division work—that is, for the aforementioned in-depth exploration of a major field of study at the upper-division level. If this
principle is honored and internalized, the methodologies for the
program delivery will be appropriate and credible.

One way to guard and protect the meaning and integrity of the
academic degree is for nurse educators to get in the habit of using
terms that describe their programs rather than their students. For
example, students enrolled in an associate degree nursing program are associate degree nursing students, whether they are
licensed practical nurses or high school graduates without any
nursing background. Students enrolled in a baccalaureate nursing
program are baccalaureate nursing students, whether they are
RNs, LPNs, high school graduates, or lawyers. Terms such as
"generic program," "RN completion program," or "two-plus-two
program" tend to confuse or denigrate the meaning and value of
the academic degree being pursued.

In addition, these terms do not serve us well because they are
not understood by our colleagues in higher education or by the
public at large. For example, Webster's defines *generic* as "of,
applied to, or referring to a whole kind, class, or group"; it also
means "that which is not a trademark." It is unclear just how the
word *generic* worked its way into the language of nursing education or why it is used to describe the student who is not a nurse
or the program that admits such students. Clearly, non-nurse
students are all students. No useful purpose is served by labeling
them with terms that have no relevance. Nurse educators need
to be more consistent in describing their programs by the degree
conferred rather than by the kind of student admitted, because
the more often students hear the right descriptors about themselves, the more socialized they will become to their new role.

'A Phenomenon Whose Time Has Come'

Clarity about career mobility and all terms associated with it is
important because the burgeoning of the movement toward de-

veloping career mobility options throughout the nursing education system is undeniable and will undoubtedly continue for the
foreseeable future. Part of the impetus for a new surge of interest
in this concept occurred in 1984 when the House of Delegates of
the National Federation of Licensed Practical Nurses voted over-
whelmingly to expand their programs to a minimum of 18 months
so that an associate degree could be conferred upon completion
of the program ("NFLPN OKs 'Two Nursing Levels,' " 1984).
Other chapters in this book deal with career mobility as it relates
to the implementation of two levels of practice for nursing. But
even if none of these events were transpiring, upward mobility
for nursing would still be a phenomenon whose time has come.
    In 1979, Notter and Robey wrote:

> It is almost rhetorical to ask whether upward mobility is or
> should be possible. The entire thrust of social thought in this
> century has been toward allowing the individual to reach his
> highest potential. Even if nursing could turn back the clock
> to a time when class and role were immutable there is every
> reason to believe that this would not be in the best interests
> of the profession.

    If numbers are any indicator, the interests of the profession are
indeed being served. Between 1975 and 1984 the number of RNs
enrolled in baccalaureate programs that also admit unlicensed
people increased by 111 percent; the number of baccalaureate
programs that admit only RNs rose to a high of 170; the number
of RNs enrolled in the latter programs almost quadrupled; and
the number of RNs graduating from baccalaureate programs increased from 3,763 to over 10,000 annually (Rosenfeld, 1986). Although the statistics on the numbers of licensed practical nurses
enrolling in associate degree nursing programs are less readily
available, it is worthy of note that a recent survey of the 18 associate degree nursing programs in Tennessee showed that all
programs had advanced placement procedures for LPNs, the
number of LPNs enrolling in these programs is increasing, and
nearly 600 LPNs had earned associate degrees in Tennessee in
the last five years ("Tennessee Nurses' Association Survey," 1986).
Clearly, licensed nursing personnel are moving upward through
the nursing education system.
    From a review of the literature and an analysis of the trends
developing in nursing education, it is safe to say that career mobility at the associate degree and baccalaureate levels in nursing

is here to stay and that several successful and effective models have been developed to accommodate students in flexible ways without compromising program quality. Since the focus of this book is titling and licensure, this chapter does not treat questions of articulation and career mobility related to graduate nursing education in detail. Few graduate nursing programs currently admit unlicensed students, although there is evidence that the number of such programs may be increasing. However these programs develop, they will be educationally sound and highly credible if those responsible for them maintain, protect, and preserve the value and commonly understood and accepted meaning of the master's and doctoral degrees by creating programs that operationalize an authentic philosophy of graduate education. Or, to put it another way, career mobility and program integrity need not and must not be mutually exclusive. Once the meaning and value of the academic degree that is conferred upon completion of a nursing program is recognized and internalized, a variety of valid and useful models for program delivery at all levels will emerge that will simultaneously enhance program quality while being responsive to students' needs and interests.

CAREER MOBILITY FOR FACULTY

Just as many students enter, exit, reenter, and reexit nursing programs in large numbers, so also do many faculty members move periodically from one institution of employment to another. In that process, faculty members sometimes find themselves teaching in a program quite different from the one they left. For our purposes, the phenomenon known as faculty mobility may be defined simply as the process of transition from one nursing faculty position to another. The transition may be lateral—for example, from one baccalaureate program to another—or vertical—such as from an associate degree to a graduate program, a diploma to an associate degree program, a baccalaureate to an associate degree program, and so forth. While adjustment to a new position is probably always somewhat stressful, these stresses can be minimized and the success rate for career changes can be enhanced if the process is better understood.

Although hard comparative data are difficult to obtain, it seems reasonable to hypothesize that nursing faculty may be more mobile than faculty from some other disciplines. There are several factors that support this belief. First, the job market for nursing faculty has expanded enormously. The number of nursing programs in the United States, excluding LPN programs, increased from 1,264 in 1968 to 1,556 in 1984, and the number of full-time faculty employed in these programs increased from slightly less than 15,000 to more than 20,000 during the same period. The number of full-time faculty employed in baccalaureate and higher degree programs more than doubled during that time, and the number of faculty employed in associate degree programs quadrupled (Gothler, 1986). A second factor to support the existence of high mobility among nursing faculty members is the continual upgrading of the academic and experiential requirements for faculty appointments in various types of nursing programs. For most if not all associate degree programs, faculty members must now hold a master's degree in nursing. A master's degree in nursing is an absolute requirement for all baccalaureate and higher degree programs, and a doctorate or evidence of progress toward that degree is increasingly expected; for some baccalaureate and higher degree programs, the doctoral degree is a requirement for employment. Since the supply of nursing faculty members prepared at these levels is below the demand, those who hold these credentials are actively and aggressively recruited and are highly marketable. Consider, for example, the fact that despite a significant increase in the number of nurses who hold graduate degrees in nursing, in 1984 there were still 259 full-time nursing faculty members teaching in baccalaureate nursing programs who held the BSN as their highest academic credential. There were nearly 1,300 baccalaureate-prepared full-time faculty members teaching in associate degree programs that same year. And, despite vigorous recruitment and educational efforts, only one in five faculty members teaching in baccalaureate or graduate nursing programs in 1984 was doctorally prepared (Gothler, 1986).

A third factor that probably makes nursing faculty more mobile is the predominance of women in the profession. Unmarried or single-parent nursing faculty members are, as a group, probably more mobile than married nurse faculty members. That phenomenon is changing, however, and in any event, male or female married nursing faculty members may relocate either to advance their own careers or because their spouse has an opportunity for upward career mobility.

The literature yields some helpful insights about making an effective transition to the nursing faculty role (Conway & Glass, 1978; Fitzpatrick & Heller, 1980; Infante, 1986; Lenz & Waltz, 1983; Sorensen, Van Ort, & Weinstein, 1985). Most of the information, however, is related to how one can move successfully from a graduate student or nursing practice role to the role of a nurse educator. Very little has been written about transitional problems arising from moving from the teaching role in an associate degree or diploma program to the role of a faculty member in a baccalaureate program or about any of the other career moves that nurse educators are now making in large numbers. Since the phenomenon of faculty mobility is occurring with increasing frequency, it is timely to attempt to identify approaches that will make these career changes more positive and effective.

The key word used in the role transition literature is *socialization*, which the dictionary defines as "the process of forming associations or of adapting oneself to them; especially the process whereby an individual acquires the modifications of behavior and the values necessary for the stability of the social group of which he is or becomes a member." From this definition one might conclude that, in order to be successful in any new role, one must demonstrate the behaviors and internalize the values that are commonplace within the social group that one is joining. At face value that seems simple enough. But behaviors and values are not automatically, thoughtlessly, or easily changed. Behaviors and values arise from a base of knowledge and experience that develops over time with input from a variety of sources. In order for the transition to be smooth and successful, therefore, several important processes should be initiated.

The first is to determine that there is a "good match" between the academic and experiential background of the prospective faculty member and the faculty group he or she is considering joining. Specifically, it is probably not wise to even apply for a faculty position at an institution where almost everyone is better prepared than the applicant. If 75 percent of a nursing faculty employed at a college that offers BSN, MSN, and PhD nursing programs is doctorally prepared and all have had at least three years of teaching experience at one of those levels, it is difficult to imagine that a master's prepared nurse with no prior teaching experience at the baccalaureate or higher degree level will be effectively socialized into that particular faculty group. The knowledge and experiential base from which the group's behaviors and values have evolved is beyond that which this applicant can bring to the setting. To state the problem another way, this prospective faculty member does not have enough in common with the group he or she would like to join. The difference between the applicant and the reference group is such that no orientation program, no matter how comprehensive, can eliminate it.

But even when the academic and experiential differences are minimal, absent, or in favor of the prospective faculty member, a number of activities should be initiated to facilitate the correct career decision and to make the transition as smooth as possible. It is of critical importance, for example, that the prospective faculty member become familiar and conversant with the mission, goals, and priorities of the parent institution. Obviously, the mission of a community college is quite different from the mission of an academic health sciences center. It is important to understand the institutional mission because understanding is prerequisite to acceptance and internalization, two phenomena that must occur if the role transition is to be successful.

Once an individual is comfortable and enthusiastic about participating in the achievement of the institution's mission, the next step is to understand and internalize the philosophical belief system that undergirds the nursing program. Since program objectives, the curriculum itself, the teaching-learning strategies utilized for program delivery, and the types of students suited for the program all emerge from the program's philosophy it is imperative that the prospective faculty member be well informed about and philosophically compatible with all of these factors. This is important not only for effective transition or successful socialization, but also to protect the integrity of the program and to ensure its growth.

The necessary new knowledge base can be acquired and the new value system internalized through taking additional courses, attending workshops or seminars, reviewing and absorbing relevant literature, reading and assimilating information and materials published by the employing institution, discussing unanswered issues or questions with appropriate institutional representatives, or a combination of several of these methods. Whatever methods are utilized, it is crucial that philosophical and programmatic compatibility be achieved so that the role transition is smooth, the socialization process is successful, and the program is enriched rather than hampered.

CONCLUSIONS

Students in large and increasing numbers are moving upward through the nursing education system. This movement is appropriate, will strengthen the nursing profession, and should be facilitated by nurse educators. A wide variety of models for program delivery are currently in use. As long as these models ensure program quality and protect the integrity of the degree, they are legitimate and acceptable.

As faculty members continue to upgrade and improve their collective academic credentials and as the numbers of associate degree, diploma, and baccalaureate programs continue to fluctuate, the movement of nursing faculty members from one kind or level of nursing program to another will probably increase. These career moves will be more successful and the process of transition to the new role will be less stressful if faculty members bring to their new employment setting the academic credentials stipulated for the position, the appropriate expertise to assume the new role, and the internalization of the philosophy and mission of the parent institution and of the nursing program.

REFERENCES

Allison, S. E., Balmat, C. S., Keheley, P. C., Shoptaw, M. S., Anderson, B., Hinton, P. A., & King, F. E. (1984). Externship programs: The Mississippi model. *Nursing Outlook, 32,* 207–209.

Boyle, R. E. (1972). Articulation: From associate degree through master's. *Nursing Outlook, 20,* 670–672.

Bullough, B. (1972). You can't get there from here: Articulation in nursing education. *Journal of Nursing Education, 11*(4), 4–10.

Bullough, B. (1979). The associate degree: Beginning or end? *Nursing Outlook, 27,* 324–328.

Burnside, H. (1969). Practical nurses become associate degree graduates. *Nursing Outlook, 17*(4), 47.

Conway, E. E., & Glass, L. K. (1978). Socialization for survival in the academic world. *Nursing Outlook, 26,* 424–429.

Corona, D. F. (1970). A continuous process curriculum in nursing. *Nursing Outlook, 18*(1), 46–48.

Davis, A., Shiber, S., & Allen, J. (1984). Weekend college. *Nursing Outlook, 32,* 259–263.

Directory of career mobility programs in nursing education. (1976). New York: National League for Nursing.

Drage, M. O. (1971). Core courses and a career ladder. *American Journal of Nursing, 71,* 1356–1358.

Fasano, M. A. (1976). From LVN to RN in one year. *Nursing Outlook, 24,* 251–253.

Fitzpatrick, M. L., & Heller, B. R. (1980). Sounding board: Teaching the teachers to teach. *Nursing Outlook, 28,* 372–373.

Galliford, S. (1980). Second step baccalaureate programs in nursing. *Nursing Outlook, 28,* 631–635.

Gothler, A. (1986). *Nurse faculty: Socioeconomic trends—1985.* New York: National League for Nursing.

Gross, L. C., & Bevil, C. W. (1981). The use of testing to modify curricula for RN's. *Nursing Outlook, 29,* 541–545.

Hale, S. L., & Boyd, B. T. (1981). Accommodating RN students in baccalaureate nursing programs. *Nursing Outlook, 29,* 535–540.

Hall, K. V. (1979). Current trends in the use of conceptual frameworks in nursing education. *Journal of Nursing Education, 18*(4), 26–29.

Hangartner, C. A. (1966). College credit equivalency and advanced standing. *Nursing Outlook, 14*(5), 30–32.

Infante, M. S. (1986). The conflicting roles of nurse and nurse educator. *Nursing Outlook, 34,* 94–96.

Integrity in the college curriculum: A report to the academic community. (1985). Washington, D.C.: Association of American Colleges.

Kramer, M. (1970). Credit for competency. *American Journal of Nursing, 70,* 793–798.

Laverdier, R. (1973). An accelerated nursing curriculum. *Nursing Outlook, 21,* 524–526.

Lenburg, C. B. (1975). Open curriculum: Two faces on each side of the coin. In L. Notter (Ed.), *Proceedings: Open curriculum conference II* (pp. 18–34). New York: National League for Nursing.

Lenburg, C., & Johnson, W. (1974). Career mobility through nursing education: A report on NLN's open curriculum. *Nursing Outlook, 22*(4), 265–269.

Lenburg, C. B., & Rapaport, D. S. (1979). LP/VN to RN: A program designed for you. *Journal of Practical Nursing, 39*(11), 22–24.

Lenz, E. R., & Waltz, C. F. (1983). Patterns of job search and mobility among nurse educators. *Journal of Nursing Education, 22,* 267–273.

MacLean, T. B., Knoll, G. H., & Kinney, C. K. (1985). The evolution of a baccalaureate program for registered nurses. *Journal of Nursing Education, 24*(2), 53–57.

Malkin, E. (1966). Direction of dilemma for RN's. *Nursing Outlook, 14*(5), 36–38.

Marsh, H. F., & Lasky, P. A. (1984). The professional portfolio: Documentation of prior learning. *Nursing Outlook, 32,* 264–267.

Moore, N. E. (1981). Climbing the career ladder from LP/VN to RN. *Journal of Practical Nursing, 3*(10), 45, 53–54.

NFLPN OKs "two nursing levels," 18-month curriculum for LPN's. (1984). *American Journal of Nursing, 84,* 1303, 1312, 1314.

National League for Nursing. (1970). *The open curriculum in nursing, 1970:* A statement approved by the Board of Directors, National League for

Nursing, February 1970. Reprinted in L. E. Notter & M. Robey (Eds.), *The open curriculum in nursing: Final report of the NLN open curriculum study* (p. 381). New York: National League for Nursing, 1979.

Notter, L. E., & Robey, M. C. (1979). Open curriculum practices. *Nursing Outlook, 27,* 116–121.

Reed, S. B. (1979). Part 1: The process and the plan. *Journal of Nursing Education, 18*(9), 10–25.

Rosenfeld, P. (1986). *Nursing student census with policy implications—1985.* New York: National League for Nursing.

Smailer, C. (1979). Education at large: The ladder without range. *Imprint, 26*(1), 28, 62.

Sorensen, G. (1976). Sounding board: In support of the generic baccalaureate degree program. *Nursing Outlook, 24,* 384–385.

Sorensen, G. E., Van Ort, S. R., & Weinstein, A. C. (1985). Faculty mobility in baccalaureate and higher degree nursing programs in research I and II universities. *Journal of Professional Nursing, 1,* 138–144.

Spurr, S. H. (1970). *Academic degree structures: Innovative approaches.* A general report prepared for the Carnegie Commission on Higher Education. New York: McGraw-Hill.

Stevens, B. J. (1981). Program articulation: What it is and what it is not. *Nursing Outlook, 29,* 700–706.

Styles, M. M., & Wilson, H. S. (1979). The third resolution. *Nursing Outlook, 27*(1), 44–47.

Tennessee Nurses' Association survey of nursing education programs (June 1986). Unpublished report, Tennessee Nurses' Association, Nashville, Tennessee.

Walsh, J. E. (1975). Development of open curriculum nursing programs: Approaches to administrative problems. In L. Notter (Ed.), *Proceedings: Open curriculum conference II* (pp. 35–43). New York: National League for Nursing.

Waters, V. (1976). Pressures for opening the curriculum. In M. W. Searight (Ed.), *The second step* (pp. 1–10). Philadelphia: F. A. Davis.

Wozniak, D. (1973). External degrees in nursing. *American Journal of Nursing, 73,* 1014–1018.

Zusey, M. L. (1986). RN to BSN: Fitting the pieces together. *American Journal of Nursing, 86,* 394–397.

CHAPTER 5

Transforming the Patterns of Nursing Education

Carl Miller

Nursing programs throughout the United States are in a state of transition. The recent positions related to nursing practice and education taken by the National League for Nursing and the American Nurses' Association, coupled with the ensuing interpretive statements, collaboration, speeches by staff of both organizations, panel discussions, and debates, have directed the attention of nursing educators to the changes taking place in the institutional structure of nursing programs. These changes have taken a multitude of forms, but most of these involve redesigning the program to somehow fit in with the nationally accepted system of higher education. In some schools across the country, changes have already been made; in others, plans are being developed to make the necessary shifts to keep pace with what faculty perceive as nursing education's future direction. Regardless of the new forms these programs take, however, this chapter will argue that certain elements must be present to assure the development of high-quality, accreditable nursing education.

STATUS OF NURSING EDUCATION TODAY

It seems in retrospect that there was no better time than the years following World War II, when thousands of students flocked

67

to colleges and universities, for nursing to intensify its efforts to attain a long-proclaimed educational goal of moving into the main-stream of higher education. Emerging advances in science and technology heightened the need for a better-educated population, including those in nursing. Today, in contrast, rapid expansion followed by recent years of constricting resources and leveling enrollments have taken their toll on higher education. Both ac-commodating large numbers of ill-prepared students who entered academia as the result of open enrollment and the general decline of educational standards in the public schools have weakened the quality of academic programs.

Evidence of decline in higher education is abundant. The busi-ness community, for example, complains of difficulty in recruiting literate college graduates. Remedial programs, designed to com-pensate for lack of skills in speaking and writing the English language and in manipulating basic principles of mathematics, abound on college and university campuses. Grades have gone up and up, even as Scholastic Aptitude Test and American College Testing Program scores have gone down; and pressures on teach-ers to ease their students' paths to graduate schools have in-creased. Skepticism and decreasing public confidence concerning the quality of higher education are invited when available evi-dence suggests that colleges and universities may be awarding degrees to students who do not possess even basic academic skills.

In addition to the threat posed by increasing negative public opinion, the existence of some colleges is threatened by a decline in the annual number of high school graduates, which has dropped 12 percent since 1980–81. Many colleges have been able to offset this decline by recruiting large numbers of older students. Michael O'Keefe (cited in Benderson, 1986) reports that 660,000 more peo-ple between the ages of 22 and 34 enrolled in college in 1983 than in 1979 and goes on to say that the decline of available 18-year-olds won't hit bottom until 1992, at which time the pool will be decreased by 26 percent. O'Keefe suggests that schools which draw a greater percentage of their students from the traditional pool, such as small, private liberal arts colleges, will be the hardest hit by this trend.

As if these facts and figures did not pose enough challenge to nurse educators in their efforts to reach long-awaited goals in higher education, there is a growing sentiment that opposes the desire of nursing and other health-related professions to require higher, more costly degrees for entry into the profession. A report prepared by a commission of the Southern Regional Educational

Board recommended that governors and state legislators should "oppose moves by organizations of medical professionals to raise the minimum degree requirements for entry into their professions." The report continues:

> If certain professions are pressing for higher academic levels of education, state governments must assure that employers and the public really require such advanced levels of education. . . . State officials must be prepared to resist "degree creep" by professions and educators when it is unwarranted [Jaschik, 1986].

In view of the essence of this report, one feels compelled to ask, must nursing, which came through the back door of colleges and universities, now defend its right to bring the whole of nursing education into the parlor where it has achieved a rightful place?

Movement of the educational system for nursing into the mainstream of higher education is beginning to have an ancient and perhaps at times a monotonous ring. Major studies released over the past 50 years have proclaimed and advanced the virtues of movement in this direction. Perhaps, as noted earlier, there were times in nursing's past when such a transition could have been accomplished through careful planning and orderly implementation. Those times have now passed, and this transition is occurring rapidly and randomly in nursing education across the country. It is understandably being approached with some hesitation, a degree of reluctance, and considerable fear by those directly involved in the process and with a mixture of reservation, suspicion, ambivalence, and in some instances, rejection by those who hold appointments in established programs. The question before nursing is how to cope with this mix of emotions in successfully resolving the dilemma that nursing has lived with and suffered from for more than 75 years as a "nonsystem" of education. Given existing conditions, how can necessary changes be made while preserving that which constitutes quality in nursing education.

Transition by definition involves passage or evolution from one form to another. Retaining what "is" does not accomplish this. Faculty who are involved in transitions in educational programs are noticeably reluctant to make a complete and thorough move, to assume all the traits and distinguishing qualities that characterize the form to which the program wishes to progress. However, successful, accreditable transitions cannot be accomplished by retaining the old forms, including (1) an organizational structure and governance that does not have education as its primary focus, (2) the essence of the former curriculum, which was preparing students for a different level of nursing practice, (3) a milieu that has a service rather than educational focus, or (4) a faculty that lacks the academic and experiential credentials requisite for teaching in institutions of higher learning. Control of the program must rest with the college or university granting the degree. Only those faculty members who meet established criteria for appointment of all college or university faculty and who have an appropriate background for meeting program goals should be appointed. The educational milieu, the curriculum, and the preservation of its integrity are the responsibility of those individuals who are appointed as faculty. The criteria for accreditation of nursing programs, as normatively derived expectations of the requisite resources and characteristic processes and outcomes judged to be indicative of quality education, should be followed as guidelines by programs in transition to ensure that the new programs they design are indeed accreditable.

ORGANIZATIONAL STRUCTURE AND GOVERNANCE

Of critical importance in the establishment and organization of a program in nursing is clearly identifying the parent institution. This is a major issue in the accreditation of programs to establish who oversees the program and to preserve its educational integrity. Within the traditional college or university setting this is a relatively simple task. In the case of a program that stands alone, however, owned and operated by an institution or corporation whose primary goal and function is health care delivery, or a program under similar control offered collaboratively with a college or university, the task of identifying the parent institution is not so simple.

A basic principle in identifying institutional parenthood is that the parent must possess the traits and characteristics it wishes to transmit to the offspring. A health care delivery institution cannot easily develop a reputation for possessing the traits and characteristics of an academic program, and therefore, is faced with some difficulty in declaring itself the parent of an offspring it wishes to have recognized as an academic professional program. Collaboration with an institution of higher learning in the development of a program makes it easier to identify an appropriate parent for a program. In this instance, growth and development of the program's educational quality logically rests with the institution that has education as its primary goal.

In the final analysis, legitimate parenthood for an academic program requires the establishment of an organizational structure and governance controlled and operationalized by recognized educators representing diverse disciplines that bring together the faculty, curriculum offerings, and resources and services necessary for producing a liberally educated graduate. This is not to imply that an institution whose primary goal is health care delivery cannot be involved in education or that education should be removed from involvement in health care delivery. The issue is one of appropriate control for maximizing quality, whether within the educational system or the health care delivery system. Enhancement of educational quality and ensuring educational integrity does not appropriately fall within the realm of those whose primary goal is health care delivery, just as the assurance of quality health care cannot be considered appropriate responsibilities for those whose primary goal is education.

Financial support of academic programs in nursing by health care delivery institutions creates a natural tendency to expect some level of involvement in decision making and in that respect a certain degree of control. After all, as the old saying goes, "Whoever pays the piper calls the tune." Fiscal viability is obviously significant as one considers the characteristics of a quality educational program. The cost of assuring that viability is too great, however, if the responsibility for educational decisions and program implementation is sacrificed or in any way altered in an effort to obtain the assurance of funding.

MILIEU

One hundred years ago, John Henry Newman recognized the value of the educational milieu:

> When a multitude of young men, keen and open-minded, sympathetic and observant, . . . come together and freely mix with each other, they are sure to learn from one another. . . . The conversation of all is a series of lectures to each and they gain for themselves new ideas and views, fresh matters of thought and distinct principles for judging and acting [cited in Martin & Svaglic, 1960, p. 110].

Research also demonstrates that students' interactions with their teachers, their encounters with the social structure of college administration, the friendship group in which they become integrated, the values they acquire from the student culture all have an immense if not precisely measured impact on the evolution of their view of self and world, on their confidence and altruism, and on their mastery of the need for identity (Study Group on the Conditions of Higher Education in American Education, 1984).

In this period of educational transition, we can not lose sight of the struggles in which nursing has engaged to become part of the academic community and to be considered equal partners with other disciplines in the advancement of knowledge pertinent to the needs of society. Over the past 20 years, nursing has succeeded in reaching a goal pursued for over a century. In 1960, 83 percent of the new graduates were educated in hospital schools. By 1980, this trend was completely reversed: 83 percent of the new nursing graduates received their education in colleges and universities, and the trend continues (Garnick & Lewin, 1984). It is imperative that nursing protect the turf gained and guard against any transitional direction that cannot ensure the academic integrity of the nursing degrees.

These comments are not intended to imply that there is but one model for nursing education, or that such a model should be inflexible and used punitively in making decisions regarding quality. Rather, the intention is to emphasize the importance of assuring that the patterns of nursing education that emerge and that are sanctioned through peer review produce not only nurses but educated individuals who possess a broad foundation drawn from the humanities and biophysical and behavioral sciences and who can use their education to enhance themselves as individuals and as productive, influential members of society.

CURRICULUM AND THE EDUCATED NURSE

The importance of higher education in America is being proclaimed today with renewed vigor at the same time that its quality and integrity, as already mentioned, are under careful scrutiny. This concerted attention seems clearly related to the matter of how well higher education will meet the demands of the future.

As one recent report points out: "As American society has demanded a more educated work force, higher education has become not merely a preserver and transmitter of culture but an integral part of our economic progress and national well-being" (National Institute of Education, 1984). Perhaps because of the value placed on higher education, educators have expressed major concerns regarding current conditions and an urgent desire to have higher education assume the significant role expected by society. For example, in a recent report the Association of American Colleges (1985) indicated that "almost anything goes" in a college curriculum today and that "We have reached a point at which we are more confident about the length of a college education than its content and purposes." This accusation leads to the question, "Is the curriculum an invitation to philosophic and intellectual growth or a quick exposure to the skills of a particular vocation?" The report asserts that curriculum emphasizes content and neglects the essential style of inquiry on which the content is based. With declines in enrollment, the report charges, a "survival ethic" dominates the thinking of many institutions. As a result, the curriculum has given way to a marketplace philosophy that refuses to establish common expectations and norms: "It is a supermarket where students are shoppers and professors are merchants of learning. Fads and fashions, the demands of popularity and success enter where wisdom and experience should prevail" (Association of American Colleges, 1985).

This is perhaps a rather dismal portrayal of American higher education. On a more positive note, efforts are under way to maximize the potential benefit derived from higher education and thereby meet more fully the significant role expected by society. In their report of the academic community, the Association of American Colleges' (1985) committee of educators proposed that we develop a system of education "that will enable the American people to live responsibly and joyfully, fulfill their promise as individual humans and their obligations as democratic citizens." The report suggests nine experiences as essential to that kind of education. Some of them are thought of as skills, others as ways of growing and understanding; all of them are considered basic to higher education on the undergraduate level. These experiences include:

1. Inquiry: abstract logical thinking, critical analysis
2. Literacy: writing, reading, speaking, listening
3. Understanding numerical data
4. Historical consciousness
5. Science

6. Values
7. Art
8. International and cultural experiences
9. Study in-depth [Association of American Colleges, 1985]

A similar list appears in a working document issued by the American Association of Colleges of Nursing (1980) which identifies behaviors that a professional nurse should demonstrate as an educated person:

1. Write, read, and speak English clearly and effectively.
2. Think analytically and reason logically on the basis of verifiable information.
3. Use a second language, at least at an elementary level.
4. Understand mathematical concepts, interpret quantitative data, and use computers and other information technology.
5. Use knowledge from the behavioral and life sciences to understand oneself and one's relationships with other people and comprehend the nature of communities.
6. Understand the physical world and its interrelationship with human activity.
7. Understand life and time from a historical perspective and use this knowledge of the past to inform present and future behavior.
8. Understand current social, political, and economic issues and use knowledge about them to participate in their resolution.
9. Understand and appreciate cultures other than one's own.
10. Comprehend the meaning of human spirituality from the study of comparative religions, literature, philosophy, and psychology.
11. Appreciate the expressive and performing arts and the nature and usefulness of creative thought.
12. Understand the nature of human values and make ethical judgments in both personal and professional life [American Association of Colleges of Nursing, 1980].

This report also describes the faculty's contributions in the development of these behaviors:

Faculty in the fine arts, humanities, social sciences, and sciences are responsible for instructing the nursing student in the knowledge and methods of their disciplines; but faculty in nursing must guide the student in the further development and application of this knowledge. For instance, clear and literate writing must be expected and encouraged in all nursing courses, just as nursing curricula must provide continuing practice in creative and critical thinking, ethical judgment, and intercultural understanding. Arts and science faculty bear primary responsibility for the liberal education, . . . but professors of nursing must respect and model the enlightened use of that knowledge in their classrooms and in clinical settings [American Association of Colleges of Nursing, 1980].

These statements clearly indicate the requisites for those students in nursing who seek to become and who wish to be viewed by others as educated people as well as the role faculty assume in this process. Within this context, the greatest challenge that faces nursing education is preserving the experiences that are needed to develop an educated person during and following the period of transformation in the patterns of nursing education. This challenge cannot be met by simply adding courses to a curriculum that together meet the required hours for receiving a degree or by filling the ranks of faculty with people who do not have the appropriate academic and experiential credentials needed to ensure the availability of student experiences that produce educated graduates. Higher education will mean little if the degrees students seek are weakened by reduced standards, or if academic credentials are allowed to supersede the pursuit of learning and accepted definitions of quality. The possibility of creating and maintaining these standards in environments outside the traditional university or college setting has been questioned by many nurse educators.

For academic programs in nursing outside the traditional setting to move forward from the standpoint of development of an educated individual, the process of learning, and faculty, they must be able to answer the following basic questions affirmatively:

1. Are faculty educated at the graduate level in nursing, and do they possess the capacity to transmit technical and theoretical knowledge relevant to the discipline of nursing? Equally important, are faculty prepared as educators, in the broadest sense, with a perspective of higher education and do they possess the ability to develop a teaching milieu that interrelates professional and liberal education? Are faculty expected and encouraged to engage in scholarly pursuits and professional activities, and participate in the governance of the academic institution?

2. Can nursing faculty, who represent a learned profession, develop a valued association and engage in frequent and consistent dialogue with faculty from the physical, biological, and social sciences and humanities for the purpose of joining their efforts in the development of educated graduates?

3. Can the student be provided the appropriate experiences to teach her or him how to learn, synthesize, and reshape information, drawing to the fullest extent on humankind's cumulative intellect in the resolution of the dilemmas confronting it?

These questions have not been developed for the purposes of eliminating the possibility of any new, innovative, or creative program design or for concluding that certain types of programs simply will not work. Rather, these questions are intended to represent a frame of reference for weighing whether the quality of nursing education is advanced or deterred by the choices that are made in program redesign.

CONCLUSION

When faced with current health problems, advances in health care, a changing health care delivery system, and the sociopolitical forces influencing the nursing profession, it is difficult to see how there is time to agonize and debate for very long over the issue of educational patterns for nursing. There is no doubt that many institutions have to face the reality of change, and others will have to make the difficult but perhaps wise choice to close their doors. Clearly, the future will be different from the past. The advances made by nurses in institutions of higher learning must form the foundation for charting that future if nursing is to reach its full potential.

As Lysaught (1981) noted in *Action in Affirmation: Toward an Unambiguous Profession of Nursing*, there are two ways of viewing this period of transition:

An optimist reviewing the transformation of the patterning for nursing education would argue that we are halfway to our goals; a pessimist would insist that we have failed by half to reach them. An idealist would deplore the fact that more years have been consumed in the struggle to make nursing education a unified and articulated system. A realist would simply say that the hardest part of the fight is still ahead and that our efforts must be doubled and redoubled accordingly. By any measure, there is an unfinished agenda that must be addressed with determination and decisiveness. The students, in the last analysis, shall be the ones who pay for our follies or reap the benefits of our wisdom [pp. 102–103].

REFERENCES

American Association of Colleges of Nursing. (1980). *Essentials of college and university education for nursing—A working document.* Washington, DC: American Association of Colleges of Nursing.

Association of American Colleges. (1985). *Integrity in the college curriculum: A report to the academic community.* Washington, DC: Association of American Colleges.

Benderson, A. (1986). "Higher education decline and renewal." In *FOCUS.* Princeton: ACT.

Garnick, J. C., & Lewin, L. S. (1984). *Assessment of the organizational laws of the Public Health Service nursing research activities.* Washington, DC, Department of Health and Human Services.

Jaschik, S. (1986, July 2). States are urged to consider sale of hospitals and to push for changes in medical curricula. *Chronicle of Higher Education, 32*(18).

Lysaught, J. P. (1981). *Action in affirmation: Toward an unambiguous profession of nursing.* New York: McGraw-Hill.

Martin, J., & Svaglic, S. J. (Eds.). (1960). *The idea of university.* New York: Rinehart & Co.

National Institute of Education. (1984). *Involvement in learning: Realizing the potential of American higher education.* Washington, DC: National Institute of Education.

Study Group on the Conditions of Excellence in American Higher Education. (1984, October 24). Involvement in learning: Realizing the potential of American higher education. *Chronicle of Higher Education, 6.*

PART III

Service Issues

CHAPTER 6

Issues Affecting Nursing and the Delivery of Health Care

Connie R. Curran and Neale Miller

Changes in titling and licensure of nurses have the potential to affect every practicing nurse as well as those individuals who may enter the profession in the future. Moreover, the interdependence of nursing and hospitals (nurses are the largest group of hospital employees and hospitals are the largest employers of nursing) means that changes in the nursing profession will inevitably affect the delivery of health care as a whole. This chapter will examine some of the possible effects the proposed requirements for entry into practice will have on nurses, on the nursing profession, and, by extension, on the delivery of health care.

STATE-BY-STATE DIFFERENCES

Changes in titling and licensure will occur on a state-by-state basis, resulting in a variety of different titles and licenses and diminishing nurses' interstate mobility. This interstate mobility is important to nurses' career opportunities and advancement as well as to hospital staffing. Some states have traditionally produced a surplus of nurses, while other states must consistently recruit nurses. Both "importer" and "exporter" states will experience great difficulties if states develop different titles and licenses. Hospitals may discontinue their interstate recruitment activities if difficulties exist in reciprocity.

If two licensing exams exist to determine nurses' titles, the result may be two scopes of practice and two sets of job opportunities. The scope of practice is the legal basis for employment activities, so that changes in scopes of practice will dictate changes in job functions—for example, which level of nurses will be able to administer medications or serve as care managers. If states create unique practice acts, nursing practice will vary greatly from state to state. A state that allows greater autonomy and flexibility may attract a very different type of nurse than states with restrictive practice acts. Thus, hospitals, nurses, and the general public all have a deep interest in the outcomes of the titling and licensing initiatives, and the ways in which they will affect nursing and the delivery of health care.

SUPPLY AND DEMAND

One area where the outcome of the debate over licensing and titling will have a major effect is supply and demand. Changes in licensing might facilitate entry into the profession and result in an increased supply of nurses. On the other hand, if the changes are perceived as lowering nurses' status, influence, or employment opportunities, the number of people going into and staying in nursing will decrease. And this change will take place at a time when a variety of factors are altering the nature of the demand for nursing services.

In the summer of 1985, nursing journals were filled with articles on "downsizing" and "retrenchment." A year later, these same publications were describing the shortage of critical care nurses as a national problem (see, for example, "RN Shortage Suddenly Surfaces," 1986). Cycles of shortages of nurses interspersed with short periods of an adequate supply are not new. The nursing shortage of the 1950s stimulated the preparation of technical nurses in associate degree programs. In the 1960s, shortages led to the creation of unit-manager roles. The 1970s witnessed the emergence of emergency medical technicians, physician's assistants, respiratory therapists, and other nurse substitutes. Now, in the 1980s, a surplus of physicians has created a variety of possible scenarios. The cycles in the supply of nurses are occurring more rapidly, making it difficult to respond or to track the trends. Although state legislators are likely to oppose any change in licensing that will decrease the total number of nurses, all the factors contributing to the nursing shortage must be analyzed.

One such factor is the great financial duress under which today's hospitals are operating. The shift to prospective payment systems has resulted in speculation about vast numbers of hospital closures. Predictions of an oversupply of nurses first appeared along with the prospective pricing legislation. As hospitals began to decrease their inpatient occupancy, wide publicity was given to retrenchment activities. Employee layoffs were often publicized as nursing layoffs.

Prospective payment resulted in decreased length of stay and an average occupancy rate in 1986 of 63 percent. Despite this decreased occupancy rate, however, the nurse-patient ratio has increased significantly. In 1985, 85 nurses were employed per 100 patients, compared to only 50 nurses per 100 patients in 1975 ("ANA '86—Securing the Future," 1986). Increased patient acuity has resulted in more nurses caring for fewer, sicker patients. This increase in nurse-patient ratios has contributed to the current nursing shortage.

Two other factors also responsible for this shortage are decreases in federal funding and declining college enrollments. The Nurse Training Act was passed to combat the nurse shortage of the 1960s and to meet the needs of the Great Society. Federal funds were appropriated to foster nursing education and were made available to students as scholarships, traineeships, and loans. Colleges received funds for buildings, equipment, faculty training, and curriculum development. This support reached a peak of $150 million in 1974 and dropped to $46 million in 1982 (Feinberg, 1986). As government funding has decreased, however, so have the number and quality of students admitted to nursing education programs. The absence of federal funds makes financing nursing education difficult for students and academic institutions.

In fact, the number of applicants to all types of nursing education programs has dropped consistently since 1983. The increasing numbers of women who are pursuing traditionally male-dominated fields is frequently cited as a reason for this move away from nursing. The status, pay, and working conditions available in fields such as law and business make it difficult to recruit students to nursing. Moreover, the end of the "baby-boom" generation has resulted in a smaller pool of applicants for all higher education. Now, even highly regarded colleges and universities have had to step up recruitment and develop innovative tactics.

Nor does the effectiveness of aggressive recruitment stop with academia. One Pennsylvania hospital instituted an on-site child care center as a recruitment incentive. This cost-effective advertising device became the primary focus of the hospital's recruitment efforts (Midei & Sanchez, 1984). If partially subsidized on-site child care could be included with other alternatives in a cafeteria-type benefits package, local nurses with young children might more readily be lured back to work. Such an incentive could also provide a competitive edge to one nursing department in a community with many hospitals.

Options such as this must be remembered as nurses analyze long-term solutions to the problems of supply and demand. It has been projected that by the year 2000 there will be a shortage of 600,000 baccalaureate and graduate degree-prepared nurses, while there will be an oversupply of 500,000 technical nurses. Planned educational remapping will be necessary to ensure an adequate supply of professional nurses who are prepared to deal creatively with rapid changes and future technological realities (Styles & Holzemer, 1986). This can happen only if nurses with many different backgrounds and priorities are willing to compromise on some long-held positions to reach a consensus. The credibility of the nursing profession as a whole and its ability to maintain some semblance of self-determination will be influenced by its response to projections of future needs.

NURSING AS A CAREER CHOICE: CHANGING OUR IMAGE

Proposed changes in the titling and licensure of nurses have the potential for both positive and negative effects on nurse recruitment and retention. A thorough analysis of factors involved in career choice as well as retention of nurses in the profession is necessary. As nursing defines new scopes of practice and new employment opportunities, it may motivate individuals to turn toward or away from the profession.

The media image of nursing is one factor that has a negative impact on nurse recruitment and retention. The research of Kalisch and Kalisch (1983a) reveals that the media portrays nurses as angels, mothers, physicians' handmaidens, sexually promiscuous, and cold-hearted. Nurses, in contrast, perceive themselves as patient advocates, patient educators, caregivers, coordinators, and researchers. The influence of the media is a major reason for the great discrepancy between the public image and the self-image.

The print and broadcast media have a tremendous impact on the ideas and opinions of most people in this country. Ninety-eight percent of all American homes have at least one television, which is operating approximately six and one-half hours a day (Kalisch & Kalisch, 1982). Most homes subscribe to at least one newspaper and one or more magazines. Over 90 percent of all automobiles have radios, and approximately the same percentage of homes have radios. Billions of visits to movies take place each year. The media bombard Americans in their homes and cars, during work, and in their leisure hours. The media serve to educate, inform, evaluate, and entertain us. And these influential media are perpetuating negative stereotypes of nursing (Kalisch & Kalisch, 1983a). Yet, the media are not intentionally maligning nursing; they are presenting what they believe is true. Nursing can counteract these stereotypes by presenting the media with information that describes nursing accurately. Kalisch and Kalisch (1985) describe several approaches that nurses and the nursing profession can take to utilize the media to promote a positive image of the profession.

Nursing is a heterogeneous profession. Nurses work in a variety of settings with a variety of individuals and families. It is not necessary to project any single image; it is imperative, however, to project a positive image. We must convey to consumers the facts that nurses are caregivers, coordinators of other health team members, patient advocates, and health educators. They are the largest group of employees in most health care institutions. Nurses spend more time caring for the ill than any other professional group. Their education and experience are a rich resource for the general public. Nurses have vast expertise to assist consumers to maintain health and prevent illness. Sharing health-related information with the public will project an accurate and professional image of nursing.

Individual and group efforts can promote a more positive image of nursing. In the early 1950s, the American Medical Association formed a group to work with the media, which has been very effective in preventing the media from projecting negative images of physicians (Kalisch & Kalisch, 1983b). Nursing can be equally effective. Media committees should be organized in hospitals, schools of nursing, and in local, state, and national nursing organizations (Curran, 1985). At a time when the entire system of nursing is in turmoil over titling issues, we run the risk of doing ourselves even greater damage through public exposure of these conflicts. It is even more important at this time to be active in working with the media to strengthen nursing's image.

IMPACT ON MINORITIES

Nursing must also examine the impact proposed licensing changes will have on minority group members, who traditionally have been underrepresented in nursing. Elementary, high school, and college educators have all lamented the poor representation of minority students on the nation's campuses and in its classrooms. According to recently published data (American Nurses' Association, 1985), members of minority groups make up approximately 10 percent of currently employed registered nurses and close to 20 percent of employed LPNs. Bezold and Carlson (1985) note that, with the exception of dietetics, practical nursing is "the major field of skilled employment for the black woman." Like other LPNs, this group faces a shrinking employment market, and may need to be encouraged to return to school for associate degrees.

There have been attempts in the past to recruit greater numbers of minority members into nursing. Those who resist the baccalaureate entry proposal cite its impact on minority members, claiming that a BSN is inaccessible to minorities. Currently, associate degree programs are financially more accessible to all potential nurses, whether they are from minority groups or not. Nearly 90 percent of associate degree education is publicly funded (subsidized by federal, state, or local taxes), while only 50 percent of baccalaureate education is underwritten by public support (American Nurses' Association, 1985). Nevertheless, the representation of minorities in baccalaureate programs is greater than that in associate degree or diploma programs. In 1983–84, of the 37,323 students admitted to baccalaureate programs 14.7 percent were members of minority groups, and minority students represented 11.3 percent of 23,107 graduates of baccalaureate nursing programs (National League for Nursing, 1986).

Public funding for support of academically qualified but financially disadvantaged students in BSN programs can do more to encourage qualified minority students to select a BSN program than any amount of rhetoric. We need to impress legislators with the potential benefit to the health care consumer of funding programs that can produce the qualified practitioners the future demands, regardless of their color of ethnic background.

Speaking as a black nurse, Maryland (1986) argues in support of the proposed changes requiring the baccalaureate degree. Keeping outdated programs alive in the name of fairness to minorities is not fairness, it is discrimination, she states. She advocates lobbying for more affirmative action scholarships and loan programs for four-year nursing programs. She also suggests developing procedures to ease the transition from existing associate degree programs with an articulated 2 + 2 model curriculum.

EDUCATION-SERVICE COLLABORATION

Historically, nursing has provided an opportunity for upward mobility to children of immigrants as well as indigenous, middle-class young women. It still provides that option for some. However, many more career options now exist for traditional high school graduates. Nursing must become more creative and competitive if it is to attract a wider range of qualified applicants who can successfully complete the baccalaureate degree and make a commitment to a flexible and rewarding career.

The primary requirement for any positive solution to the problems facing nursing is close collaboration between nurse educators and nurse executives, with input from consumer groups. One concern of that collaborative effort must be the hundreds of thousands of nurses currently functioning in hospitals and other health care settings who will continue to feel discounted, threatened, and devalued by the proposal to institute the baccalaureate degree as the entry level for professional nursing practice. The need for educators to provide accessible and creative articulation programs for current associate degree and diploma graduates cannot be overstated. As Jacquelyn Kinder (1985), president of the National League for Nursing, has stated, "We recognize that educational mobility is the most essential factor in achieving our goal."

Many excellent programs currently exist, but finding them and replicating their positive qualities is difficult. Employers can facilitate educational mobility with creative scheduling options, tuition reimbursement, scholarship aid packages, and resource people who can help employees sort through the various existing options—whether local programs or credible self-paced programs.

ECONOMIC FACTORS

Making predictions about the economic effects of changes in titling and licensure is difficult, since the definition of scope of practice and how it is translated into employment roles will determine the economic outcomes. For example, if only baccalaureate-prepared nurses are permitted to perform functions such as administration of medication and discharge planning, with less than 25 percent of RNs possessing the BS degree, a severe shortage of professional nurses could result. In most professions, a shortage of personnel leads to salary increases. Previous shortages in nursing, however, have resulted in the utilization of personnel pools and temporary employees as well as accelerated turnover rates. Clearly, recruitment and retention activities necessitated by these shortages will also have economic costs.

"Grandfathering," or allowing current practitioners to maintain their existing status, is frequently associated with proposals related to nurse titling and licensure. The specifics of which group of workers will be grandfathered into which level of nursing vary among proposals, as do the development of specific criteria for grandfathering. The grandfathering issue is complex and raises a number of questions. Should there be proficiency testing for grandfathering? What should the time frame be? How will grandfathering affect the approximately one-half million inactive nurses? The answers to these questions will directly affect large numbers of nurses and consequently the hospitals in which they practice.

The ability of organized nursing to secure direct reimbursement has numerous economic consequences. If one level of nurse has the ability to receive reimbursement and the other does not, certain types of employers may hire only those nurses who can receive reimbursement. It is conceivable that home care, ambulatory care, and outpatient services will be provided exclusively by the type of nurse that is eligible for reimbursement. If such an arrangement resulted in patient services that are less costly, both the patient and the health care delivery system could reap economic benefits.

Some feel that the proposed changes in licensure for nurses could put nurses into economic competition with physicians. Organized medicine's response to proposed changes in nursing scopes of practice may vary from state to state. If physicians feel that changes could make nurses their economic competitors, they will attempt to block the proposals. If the proposals are perceived as having positive consequences for organized medicine, they will be supportive. Nursing has a long history of fighting with medicine and losing. If the nursing profession is unable to obtain support from the various nursing factions, is it realistic to expect the support of medicine?

It is essential to ensure that the economic consequences of changes in nurse licensure are positive for patients, hospitals, nurses, and other care professionals. Because of the tremendous financial burden placed upon hospitals by prospective reimbursement, hospitals will resist all changes that create additional economic burdens. In examining alternatives, nursing must realize the potential resistance that economic issues can elicit from nurses themselves as well as from employers, regulators, and others.

SUMMARY

The issue of changes in nurse titling and licensure has numerous implications for health care delivery, the general public, and the nursing profession. The dangers are that nursing's scope of practice may be restricted, interstate mobility may be eliminated, and nurses may lose their career flexibility and status. However, opportunities exist to expand scope of practice, broaden career options, and unite nurse educators, administrators, and employers. The issue of nurse titling and licensure has the potential to move our country's largest group of health care professionals to serve the American public in new roles and new environments.

REFERENCES

American Nurses' Association. (1985). *Facts about nursing 84–85*. Kansas City, MO: American Nurses' Association.

ANA '86—securing the future. (1986). *American Journal of Nursing, 86* (7), 833–836.

Bezold, C., & Carlson, R. (1986). Nursing in the 21st century: An introduction. *Journal of Professional Nursing, 2* (1), 2–9.

Curran, C. (1985). Shaping an image of competence and caring. *Nursing & Health Care, 6*(7), 371–373.

Feinberg, L. (1986, August 11). Area nursing schools seek cure for decreasing enrollment. *Washington Post*, 1.

Kalisch, B., & Kalisch, P. (1983a). Anatomy of the image of the nurse: Dissonants and ideal models. In C. A. Williams (Ed.), *Image-making in Nursing*. Kansas City, MO: American Academy of Nursing.

Kalisch, B., & Kalisch, P. (1985). Good news, bad news and no news: Improving radio and TV coverage of nursing issues. *Nursing & Health Care, 6*(5), 255–260.

Kalisch, B., & Kalisch, P. (1983b, January). Improving the image of nursing. *American Journal of Nursing, 83*, 50.

Kalisch, B., & Kalisch, P. (1982, February). Nurses on prime-time television. *American Journal of Nursing, 82,* 264.

Kinder, J. S. (1985). Charting nursing's future (Editorial). *Nursing & Health Care, 6*(10), 519.

Maryland, M. (1986, July). Personal view: Separate but not equal. *Action on Issues* (Illinois Nurses' Association), 4.

Midei, E. L., & Sanchez, P. M. (1984, Fall). Using market research to estimate market potential and feasibility: The case of child care centers as a recruiting tool. *Health Marketing Quarterly,* 105–113.

National League for Nursing. (1986). *Nursing student census with policy implications—1985.* New York: National League for Nursing.

RN shortage suddenly surfaces in many states; Hospitals scramble to hire critical care nurses. (1986). *American Journal of Nursing 86*(7), 851–861.

Styles, M., & Holzemer, W. (1986). Educational remapping for a responsible future. *Journal of Professional Nursing,* 64–68.

CHAPTER 7

Nursing Practice in the Health Care Organization of the Future

Tim Porter-O'Grady

It may be redundant to suggest that there are many major and significant changes occurring in the health care industry. These changes appear to be paralleling the major social transformations being experienced in our nation and, indeed, in the world. Nursing, as a part of the health care delivery system, is feeling the impact of this social change—and nowhere is this change more strongly felt than in the health care institutions where today's nursing is primarily practiced. But, just as nursing is undergoing change, so are the institutions in which nurses work.

Since the introduction of the prospective payment system, diagnosis related groups (DRGs), and other fundamental cost-controlling strategies, much has changed in the hospital. Tighter controls over spending, more efficient utilization of resources, more clearly defined roles, a stronger relationship between cost and delivery of care, tighter capitalization of growth and expansion, and a renewed interest in establishing fiscal responsibility are central characteristics of the delivery of health care services today.

In the midst of all the constraints that appear to be operating in the social, political, and health care environment, nurses are attempting to offer a continuum of nursing care services. However, it is becoming increasingly difficult for nurses to maintain a predefined level of quality at a time when costs attendant to that quality are escalating. Practicing nurses are finding that institutional responses to the externally mandated changes are having a direct impact on their ability to practice nursing and to render quality clinical care. In the face of this complex situation, nursing administrators are trying to ensure the survival of their nursing organizations and maintain a defined level of quality with a contracting pool of financial resources.

At the same time, a demand exists for creative strategies and alternative services that can compensate for the decline in demand for inpatient hospital services that has resulted from the decrease in the funds available to pay for those services. Institutional administrators have developed new focuses as a result of hospitals' changing strategies for confronting the social, political, and economic changes influencing the institutional delivery of health care services.

Another major consideration having an impact on the industry as a whole has been the response from the private sector to government's decreasing interest in funding health care services. Private industry and business strategies have become an essential corollary to the operational processes currently being undertaken by hospitals. Since hospitals have not historically been good business enterprises, this change of emphasis and character in organizing and managing health care services has had a dramatic impact on the context and systems within which nursing care is being delivered today and on planning for delivery in the future. Because of the influence of business competition on hospitals and the industry as a whole, new forms of organizational strategies and relationships are being established as well as new frameworks for delivering care. These new forms demand unique and individual responses not previously conceived of by health care practitioners.

Nursing is in a key position to participate fully in this major transition in the social, economic, and delivery aspects of health care, but we must be able to anticipate future demands. No doubt, in the future, as in the past, nurses will be asked to fulfill many roles in delivering health care services that have not yet been invented but for which nurses are uniquely qualified. The breadth and depth of nursing education, based in a health and generative context rather than focused on illness and disease, uniquely prepares nurses to assume responsibilities in a broad range of new services—from preventive, interventive, maintenance, and therapeutic processes to complex illness and terminal care.

THE CORPORATE STRUCTURE

In keeping with the new business orientation and the development of operational strategies that decentralize health care services, institutions are beginning to restructure within a corporate format. Governing boards are being reorganized, and executive levels of management are beginning to operate within a corporate context. The hospital is being divided into several corporate entities, with each entity or division having responsibilities, obligations, and processes for the delivery of its services. The corporate executive body is becoming increasingly responsible for the establishment of policy, direction, and the review and approval of the financial and service mandates of the corporate board. Each corporate entity or division assumes individual responsibility for its role in fulfilling the defined corporate goals within the framework of the services and functions that are the work of that corporate segment.

As this corporate structure becomes a more common, more refined, and more acceptable mode of operation, the role of each of the corporate divisions in providing its own unique services will become even more focused and specialized. Within the corporate framework, each of the divisions will define its own parameters for work, staffing levels, financial and economic circumstances, and the outcomes it will produce as its contribution to the overall corporate goals. Each division will stand alone and compete with other divisions for resources, programs, and power within the corporation.

This kind of corporate formation, which we are just beginning to see in the multihospital systems, is becoming a standard around the nation. It will have a tremendous impact on the operational characteristics of the division of nursing in the health care institution. Nursing will no longer be a dependent piece of the organization. It will be held operationally responsible for more than defining the services it will offer. Nursing will have to articulate the parameters, provide the resources, and compete with other services, both within and outside the corporation, for programs, resources, and opportunities to participate fully in the policy and economic formation of the corporation. Changes in the industry indicate that even many small hospitals will be a part of a multiinstitutional, corporate arrangement and will play significant roles in the corporate structure in meeting a complex set of goals, objectives, and planning strategies.

THE NURSE ADMINISTRATOR

The implications of these new structures for the preparation, skills, and abilities of the nursing administrator are clear. Perhaps there will be no greater change in any nursing role than in the demands placed on this group of nurses. Nurse executives are having to develop high-level skills in corporate-level executive decision making in areas of policy, economics, marketing, business program development, and evaluation. They will also need the ability to manage a large and complex multilateral corporate division.

The responsibilities of the nurse administrator will parallel those of division administrators who are prepared at the graduate level in programs of business or health care administration in strategies of business management unique to complex organizational structures. This same kind of preparation, albeit with a nursing focus, must also become a basic part of the preparation of the nurse administrator. Integration of graduate nursing education with graduate schools of business or health services administration as a part of the educational base for the preparation of the nurse administrator should be seriously considered. Doctoral preparation in nursing and health care administration for nurse administrators in complex multihospital systems is not inappropriate for today's nurse administrator and certainly will be necessary preparation by the twenty-first century. The scope of the nursing administrator's role in today's institutions—and certainly in those of tomorrow—is beyond the ability of the nurse who has not been specifically prepared to exercise the necessary responsibilities of leadership in such a complex administrative system. Clinical preparation in nursing at the graduate level is simply not adequate to fulfill administrative roles and responsibilities in a multidivisional corporation. In short, the nursing administrator in the institutions of today and tomorrow must be specifically and adequately prepared in administrative science in order to anticipate, integrate, and facilitate the complex administrative characteristics and interactions necessary to ensure the success of a corporate self-directed division of nursing service operating in a multitude of health care environments.

THE DIVISION OF NURSING

The corporate structure of the future will demand that the divisional design of the nursing organization be self-contained and self-sustaining. The following items will become the sole responsibility of the division of nursing and the clinical and administrative nurses who comprise it:

1. The determination and specification of the services will be provided by nurses within the context of the institution. Nursing services will be self-defined and will be wholly under the control of the division of nursing.
2. Nursing care standards will be clearly described and articulated within the context of the services nurses provide. Standards of practice will be both predictive and descriptive and will be utilized to evaluate the effectiveness of the services delivered.
3. Economic, political, human, and support resources will be defined, managed, and controlled within the division of nursing. Therefore, the division of nursing will not negotiate how or how much resources will be utilized but will rather negotiate the goals anticipated for a defined fiscal period and the summary resources required to do the work of nursing directed toward meeting those goals.
4. Responsibility for clinical practice will be more clearly defined. Accountability will also be clearly delineated. Frameworks, processes, and structures will exist within the division of nursing to delineate the responsibility of the individual nurse for competence, appropriate credentialing, continuing education, and adequate preparation for the roles the nurse assumes.
5. Internal divisional structures will also be further decentralized. Each of these structures will be an independent entity, accountable solely for its own purpose, responsibilities, and functions and for justifying and clearly delineating its service parameters, processes, and outcomes agreed to through negotiation.
6. New kinds of unique, contractual arrangements will be undertaken with nurses and groups of nurses, structured and designed as part of the corporate system for delivering a broad range of services.

Clearly, these new arrangements for the organization of nursing services and new frameworks for nursing practice will require a different organizational response. A broad range of applied services will be vital to the success of nursing practice in the institution of the future.

THE ROLE OF THE PROFESSIONAL NURSE

Changes in the mechanism for licensing to establish two major nursing groups—technical and professional nurses—will have a significant impact on the way nurses are utilized in the institution. While the specifics remain as yet unclear, it is evident that more technical than professional practitioners will be available for the delivery of services to the institution. It is also clear, however, that as the preparation of professionals broadens and the academic basis for practice at the professional level deepens, the professional practitioner will either deliver or be directly responsible for a broad range of highly sophisticated clinical services.

The overall responsibility for the delivery of clinical services will be initiated, directed, and evaluated by the professional nurse. In the inpatient services, where nursing care routines are well established and well delineated, the technical practitioner would assume the broadest range of responsibility in the delivery of technical services. The responsibility for the delivery of outpatient, alternative, or other clinical services that are developed as an extension of the institution, for which a greater degree of judgment and independence would be required, would rest with the professional nurse. Since with the expansion of these types of services, there will be a greater need for practitioners with the ability to make independent judgments and assessments and to initiate care processes, a growing number of professional nurses will be required.

While it is clear that the technical nurse may assume the major responsibility for a number of technical functions, overall responsibility for both planning and implementing clinical care will rest with the professional nurse. Therefore, there will be a more direct relationship between the direction of clinical care and the actual implementation of that care within the professional practice of nursing. Thus, in the exercise of clinical functional roles within the institution, a larger number of technical practitioners will deliver care services, while outside the institution, in a more independent setting, the professional nurse will not only direct clinical care services but will be more likely to carry out those services as the primary agent with assistance from the technical practitioner.

CORPORATE RELATIONSHIPS

As already indicated, structures within the health care organization will change considerably. Accountability for the delineation of services, the articulation of those services, and the financing and policy formulation for those services will rest more consistently within the individual divisions. Because these areas of accountability will be a part of the delivery and management of the service itself within the corporate structure, each service division will have an internal corporate framework that will clearly reflect the character of the relationships in the corporate system in terms of its internal activities and its external coordinative and administrative relationships.

The nursing organization within the corporate framework will agree to fulfill specific goals and objectives, as delineated in its relationship with the institution's corporate board. It will be independently responsible for determining the services it will offer in pursuit of these goals. New types of strategies will be needed to fulfill corporate goals in the organization of the future, and the effectiveness of these strategies will depend entirely upon the kind of structural relationships and operational interactions that are developed.

Within the nursing corporate structure, it will be necessary to create an entirely new set of organizational and structural relationships to facilitate the responsibilities and functions of the participants in the organization. Traditional hierarchical relationships will not be effective in this kind of setting. They reflect neither the performance characteristics of a professional entity nor the necessity for broad-ranging, independent decision making. The new relationships must be based on peer and lateral communication and articulated interactional and functional responsibilities rather than on functional authority systems.

Nursing staff in the institutional setting of the future will be required to participate in a different way than they did under the traditional structure. They will be obligated to participate more fully in decision making and operational processes that affect their specific practice. Such participation will be required at every level, whether professional or technical, since lateral relationships and communication strategies will be essential to the effective, operational character of the organization. This means specifically that all nurses must be involved in decisions related to their responsibilities in carrying out corporate and divisional goals. Nurses in every kind of practice must be part of the processes that not only define nurses' roles but that also define the mechanism by which nurses determine their roles.

It is clear that if these characteristics become a part of the operational structure and character of the division of nursing, the structures themselves must be designed in such a way as to support this broad-based participation at all levels of nursing practice.

Peer relationships and individual accountability must be visible at every level of the organization.

GOVERNANCE

The management and governance structures that are provided within the corporate structure of the division of nursing must reflect the parallel relationships that are essential to professional practice. Since professionals relate laterally and depend on interaction and communication for delineating and carrying out their work, organized nursing activity unfolds best within a reporting structure based on serial relationships. Responsibility for such areas as practice, quality assurance, finance, and integrative governance requires working collaboratively with one's colleagues.

Since collaborative strategies, interaction, collective decision making, and integrative problem solving are key characteristics of this kind of organization, skills and abilities in those areas must obviously be a part of the talents of the nursing participants. Clearly, organizations must undertake transitional developmental activities to ensure that their participants are able to exercise their new collaborative and professional responsibilities and to integrate these processes into the ongoing functioning of the organization. Because the organization depends on each practitioner's full participation, quick orientation to and integration into the organization's activities will be an essential characteristic of beginning practice in the organization of the future. Thus, undergraduate nursing programs at both the technical and professional levels must prepare practitioners to operate successfully in a corporate environment of shared governance. Transitional academic programs preparing the professional and to some extent the technical practitioner will have to include collective, professional, collaborative skills as a major part of the nurse's skill base, even at the level of a beginning practitioner.

The role of the nursing administrator and the management team will be significantly altered in this new organizational structure. The management team actualizes many of the roles commonly identified with the executive branch of governments: facilitating, integrating, and ensuring that the decisions of the elected professional body are enacted appropriately, communicated throughout the nursing organization, delineated where necessary, and applied as appropriate in fulfilling nursing's work. This role of facilitator and integrator demands a different mix of skills from those traditionally found in the management process. The abilities to direct, decide, lead, and control as management functions will not be as valuable in the corporate professional organization of the future as they have been in the past. However, the ability to incorporate those skills into the functional roles of every practitioner and to create the environment necessary to support this activity at the practice level will be central to the success of the nurse manager and nurse administrator.

In the future, the nurse administrator will be responsible for acting as the bridge between the external and internal forces that affect nursing practice and the achievement of nursing goals and objectives. The nursing administrator must utilize her highly developed, integrative skills to observe the marketplace, and to integrate nursing responses to the external, political, social, and economic environment. The nurse administrator must moderate internal characteristics that influence the effectiveness of the nursing organization as a working unit and a team venture. The key characteristic of the nursing administrator's role will be the ability to ensure that all the elements and components of the organization come together in an integrative, organized, and systematic way and that successful outcomes can be achieved through the processes operating in a highly parallel and participatory structure. In this role, the nursing administrator is clearly central to the success of the nursing organization.

ORGANIZED DECISION MAKING

Corporate decision making will no longer remain solely a management function in the professional organization of the future. The institutional responsibility for arriving at decisions and delineating responsibility will be a shared function of designated representatives in the various components of the organization. Thus, it is important that staff nurses who have been either elected or appointed by the nursing staff assume responsibility for the decisions that ensure that appropriate clinical practice takes place. Similarly, nursing professionals will be responsible for key decisions associated with quality assurance, budget and financing, and policy essential to carrying out the work of the division of nursing.

A central governing authority that represents the key constituents of the nursing organization assumes the responsibility for ensuring that appropriate decisions are rendered and integrated.

Representation from groups that make decisions about practice, quality assurance, education, management, governance, and other activities must be formalized in this central authority to ensure that all of the activities undertaken in the division of nursing are integrated and that problems related to the effectiveness of both structure and work processes can be identified and resolved.

The horizontal and vertical flow of information and decisions throughout the organization will also be a central characteristic of the professional organization. Since in the organization of the future, decision making will be spread over a broad base, the effectiveness of communication is key to the success of the organization, and, since effective communication is so central to the organization, the channels and structures for communication must be clearly defined.

All participants who are affected by a decision must have a clear understanding of the decision, the outcomes, and the response expected of them to ensure a coherent and appropriate continuum in the delivery of services and the fulfillment of corporate obligations. Each nurse must be able not only to understand and define her role but also to identify her relationship to the organization and to the goals she is expected to fulfill. Insofar as she has been represented in defining both goals and work processes, she must be held accountable for the services that she renders and the effectiveness of those services in the environment and with the publics she is expected to serve. In the corporate organization of the future, we can no longer expect nurses to perform with a high degree of facility without the adequate information, resources, and tools to undertake their full nursing obligations. We cannot ask for a defined level of accountability without first obtaining understanding, acceptance, and full participation in the delineation of that accountability and the responsibility associated with the organization's decisions.

Peer processes then become central to the ability of each participant to relate to other participants in the collective fulfillment of nursing corporate goals and objectives. Peer relationships and responsibility and an organizational design that promotes and facilitates this interaction will be essential characteristics of the nursing organization of the future. Success will be measured by the ability of nursing staff to consult with each other, to make judgments together, to deliberate and make decisions that support each other, to communicate across service boundaries in the organization, and to challenge systems, directions, and processes in order to fully understand and be incorporated into their operational roles. When control mechanisms must be instituted, the practicing nursing staff must have a clear understanding of the framework within which such rules operate, the constraints and possibilities with which they practice, and the support and resources they have available to fulfill the obligations of their role. This nursing corporate entity, articulating for itself the mechanisms through which its goals will be fulfilled, will need the full compliance and consensus of the practitioners who will be responsible for assuring that goals get met. Clearly, then, a significant alteration in the systems, supports, and relationships will be essential to ensure success in the work of this new organizational structure.

'PRIVILEGING' AND THE NURSE'S RESPONSIBILITIES

It should be clear that hiring and credentialing of nurses in the type of participatory, laterally structured organization that has been described here will differ significantly from traditional practices in a management-dominated organization. Participation in decision making is expected at all levels of the organization. The organization's expectations of the nurse must be clearly defined, carefully structured, and agreed to at the outset as a part of the obligation of the practitioner in the setting in which she is seeking privileges.

It is important to differentiate the notion of "privileging" from that of "hiring" in a setting where professionals have an opportunity to exercise the judgment, role, and responsibility associated with professional practice. The institution that provides an environment for the practitioner to practice fully, exercising independent nursing judgment, should certainly be viewed as a privileged setting for the practitioner. When such activity is viewed within a professional context, the definition and processes associated with integrating the nurse into the organizational structure need to be significantly different. Because the professional character of nursing practice is reflected in the organization through its expectations of the nurse, it is the obligation of the nurse to indicate that she is capable of assuming the duties and responsibilities of a professional. It is not the obligation of the professional organization to ensure that its practitioners are competent and fully invested in their practice. Rather, it is the responsibility of the professional to assure her clients, her peers, and the agency that she is capable of fulfilling the requirements of her professional practice.

In the "privileging" process, the practitioner must indicate to the institution that she has a valuable and viable service to offer for which she has been prepared and that fits the needs of the institution. The applicant's preparation, skill mix, ability, service experience, and personal characteristics must lend themselves to the specific nursing role she hopes to assume in the corporate organizational structure. The role itself describes specified functions, relationships, and responsibilities. The applicant must be aware of these characteristics and must be able to give to the institution and her peers evidence that she is capable of integrating into the organization and fulfilling the obligations being asked of her as privileges are extended to her by her peers.

The "privileging" mechanism changes the locus of control in the organization from the institution and management to the individual practitioner. In the corporate model of the future, the practitioner will be required to give evidence through her clinical practice, the quality assurance program, and peer review systems that her practice and participation in the corporate process is consistent with the standards and goals established within the nursing care system. This difference in focus is both significant and valuable, and permits an integration between the system and the individual professional practitioner. The primary obligation for practice and assurance of performance rests with the practitioner, and the fundamental obligation for the integrating practice in the provision of nursing service and assuring the quality of those services rests with the corporate entity. This mutuality between organization and nurse provides, within the corporate framework, an opportunity for both complementarity and consistency between process and outcome.

It should be clear that licensure itself will not be the major consideration in reviewing a candidate's credentials and fit with the institution. Other factors that relate to the individual's aptitude for independent practice, corporate responsibility, peer relationships, and interactive skills, will be equally important considerations. The ability to participate fully in one's own practice will necessarily be a key component of the role of the nurse in an institutional setting. Since nursing will be more focused and clearly defined in a multitude of practice areas, the ability to commit oneself to practice as a career choice will be an essential characteristic of the individual who chooses to offer nursing services at either a technical or professional level.

In addition to practice responsibilities, the nurse will have corporate responsibilities in the institution. It will not be sufficient to deliver good nursing practice without fulfilling obligations to peers and to the corporate nursing organization. The nurse will participate fully in the governance and structural activities of the organization, as well as in practice and clinical activities. Within the corporate setting, the nurse has a responsibility to participate with peers in making major decisions affecting her practice and the clinical environment. She will need to relate both programmatically and politically with other disciplines and with the management team. The professional nurse will interact with others in relation to practice considerations, nursing standards, and quality assurance, and will have some role in relation to credentialing processes, by-laws, operational committees, and so forth. All of these responsibilities, when connected with the role of the practicing nurse in the clinical setting, will permit the nurse to experience the full range of professional activities associated with the delivery of clinical nursing services. Given this new scope of the nurse's obligations and responsibilities, the need to redistribute accountability and authority and reorganize structures in the organization becomes evident.

COMPETING IN THE MARKETPLACE

As the nursing organization moves with the health care delivery system into a corporate framework in the twenty-first century, it is the skills and abilities of its participants and its organizational structure that will make it a viable competitor in a new kind of marketplace. The available resources will be limited but will come from a wide variety of sources. As a result, the ability to market services, formulate strategies, and compete with others undertaking the same activities, and thus generate revenue, will be central to the success of the nursing service. No nurse, therefore, can be a member of the organization without fully participating in the goals designed to ensure financial, as well as practice viability. Since costing and charging mechanisms will be well established in the future, they will form the cost base essential to delineate appropriate payment models for remuneration of nursing services.

Unique service relationships with business, industry, other health professionals, and a wide variety of health service agencies will all be appropriate operating components of any nursing service organization, as will the ability to contract directly with others as part of a corporate strategy. The relationship of the nursing organization to the overall corporate board will be determined more by its achievement of goals and objectives than by its internal management or operating and practice mechanisms. As nursing moves into the twenty-first century, the overall corporate body will be less concerned with the internal mechanics utilized to achieve success than the outcomes for the corporation as a whole.

SUMMARY

In conclusion, it should be clear to the practicing nurse as well as management and other nursing leaders that the nursing organization of the future will have changed. The corporate reorganization of hospitals and other health care institutions today is the precursor of the major reorientation of structures that will become the routine frameworks for nursing practice in the twenty-first century.

The nurse prepared for such an environment will be required to participate fully in decisions that affect the whole range of processes operating within a corporate structure as well as in individual and collective decisions about practice in the care environment. By-laws will govern organizational relationships. Nurses, therefore, will have obligations not only to clinical practice and patient care but to operating the organization of which they are a part. They will be responsible for participating fully in defining and implementing the goals, objectives, and processes associated with providing a nursing service. Since they are invested as a constituent element of the organization, essential to its success, they will be required to participate fully in all the processes associated with the delivery of nursing services over a broad range of clinical services and options. The nurse, then, must give evidence by licensure, credentialing, and organizational participation of her commitment to her nursing organization as well as to the patient or clients she will be privileged to serve.

The corporate organization committed to the delivery of nursing service will compete in a multicorporate environment for resources and service opportunities. The ability to compete successfully with a multitude of other service organizations or corporate entities will be an essential component in delivering health care services in the future. Therefore, skills and abilities in planning, marketing, business strategy, and competition will help to ensure the viability of the nursing organization in the health care delivery process. The ability of nurses at both the professional and technical levels to confront these realities, to prepare for them now, and to commit their energy to this endeavor will truly be their measure of success.

REFERENCES

Chams, M., & Schaefer, M. (1983). *Health care organizations: A model for management.* Englewood Cliffs, NJ: Prentice Hall.

Curtin, L. (1986). Nursing in the year 2000: Learning from the future. *Nursing Management, 17*(6), 7–8.

Elbing, A. (1978). *Behavioral decisions in organizations.* London: Scott Foresman.

Gruneburg, M., & Wall, T. (1984). *Social psychology and organizational behavior.* New York: Wiley.

National Commission on Nursing Implementation Project. (1986). Unpublished working papers, Group I: Education. National Commission on Nursing Implementation Project, Milwaukee, WI.

Porter-O'Grady, T. (1986). *Creative nursing administration.* Rockville, MD: Aspen Systems Corp.

Porter-O'Grady, T., & Finnigan, S. (1984). *Shared governance for nursing.* Rockville, MD: Aspen Systems Corp.

Sandrick, K. (1986, July 5). Quality: Will it make or break your hospital? *Hospitals,* 54–58.

Appendixes

APPENDIX A

Organizational Positions on Titling and Entry into Practice: A Chronology

Denise Hartung

INTRODUCTION

The issue of educational preparation for entry into nursing practice is nearly as old as the profession itself. From nursing's onset, nursing leaders have been striving to legitimize the profession by upgrading educational standards. Esther Brown's 1948 report, *Nursing for the Future*, stated quite specifically, "We recommend that the term 'professional,' when applied to nursing education, be restricted to schools whether operated by universities or colleges, hospitals affiliated with institutions of higher learning, medical colleges, or independently; that are able to furnish professional education as that term has come to be understood by educators." The goal seemed clear and consensus of opinion within the profession easy to reach. Not so. What ensued has been the nursing profession's most unrelenting conflict.

The issue of educational preparation for entry into practice is much more than an internal professional struggle. It is a social, political, and economic issue as well. In today's health care system, with its dramatic changes in the roles of nursing and medical personnel, it is essential that nurses take decisive, sound, collec-

109

tive action to establish a truly professional status for themselves in the eyes of the public, their professional colleagues, and each other.

As nurses everywhere struggle to piece together sound information on which to base opinions about this critical issue, it is essential to take the time to look at the nursing organizations that serve as forums for the opinions of the prominent leaders of the profession and represent the collective voice of nurses. Perhaps through examining the structure of nursing organizations and the positions they have taken on this issue, consensus among nurses can be reached and a collective decision made. For here, in our nursing organizations, lies the key to resolving the issue most detrimental to nursing's professional development.

AMERICAN NURSES' ASSOCIATION

May 1960   The American Nurses' Association's Committee on Current and Long Term Goals presents a report to the ANA House of Delegates proposing a monumental goal for nursing education. This proposal is one in a series of events that would lead to ANA's eventual position on entry into practice. The proposed goal is:

> To insure that within the next 20–30 years, the education basic to the practice of nursing on a professional level, for those who then enter the field, shall be secured in a program that provides the intellectual, technical, and cultural components of both a professional and liberal education. Toward this end, the ANA shall promote the baccalaureate program so that in due course, it becomes the basic foundation for professional nursing [Henson, 1960].

1962   The ANA Board of Directors in 1962 appoints a Committee on Education to pursue the newly articulated goal.

1964   The ANA House of Delegates votes that the organization will "continue to work toward baccalaureate education as the educational foundation for professional nursing practice."

December 1965   The *American Journal of Nursing* publishes the ANA's historic position paper on education for nursing. It presents the first official position of the ANA on educational preparation for nurses. The paper focuses on four separate points:

1. The education for all those who are licensed to practice nursing should take place in institutions of higher learning.
2. The minimum preparation for beginning professional nursing practice at this time should be baccalaureate degree education in nursing.
3. The minimum preparation for beginning technical nursing practice at this time should be associate degree education in nursing.
4. The education for assistants in the health service occupations should be short, intensive preservice programs in vocational education institutions rather than on-the-job training programs. ("American Nurses' Association's First Position on Education for Nursing," 1965).

ANA continues to support three categories of personnel delivering services. The position paper specifically delineates the educational expectations of all three categories of nurses— professional, technical, and assistive. It defines the scope of practice for professional and associate nurses as follows:

Professional Nursing Practice   The essential components of professional nursing are care, cure, and coordination. The care aspect is more than "taking care of"; it is "caring for" and "caring about" as well. It is dealing with human beings under stress, frequently over long periods of time. It is providing comfort and support in times of anxiety, loneliness, and helplessness. It is listening, evaluating, and intervening appropriately. . . . It is assisting patients to understand their health problems and helping them to cope. It is the administration of medications and treatments. And it is the use of clinical nursing judgment in determining, on the basis of patients' reactions, whether the plan for care needs to be maintained or changed. It is knowing when and how to use existing and potential resources to help patients toward recovery and adjustment by mobilizing their own resources. . . . It is sharing responsibility for the health and welfare of all those in the community, and participating in programs designed to prevent disease and maintain health. It is coordinating and synchronizing medical and other professional and technical services as these affect patients. It is supervising, teaching, and directing all those who give nursing care. . . . It is using . . . knowledge, as well as other research findings, to improve services to patients and service programs to people.

Technical Nursing Practice Technical nursing practice is carrying out nursing measures as well as medically delegated techniques with a high degree of skill using principles from an ever-expanding body of science. . . . [It] is evaluating patients' immediate physical and emotional reactions to therapy and taking measures to alleviate distress. . . . [It] involves working with professional nurse practitioners and others in planning the day-to-day care of patients. It is supervising other workers in the technical aspects of care. Technical nursing practice is unlimited in depth but limited in scope. . . . It must be rendered, under the direction of professional nurse practitioners, by persons who are selected with care and educated within the system of higher education; only thus can the safety of patients be assured. ["American Nurses' Association's First Position on Education for Nursing," 1965, pp. 107–108].

The implications for education are explicit. Some diploma schools would begin to participate in programs with colleges or universities in the development of baccalaureate programs; others would participate with junior colleges in planning for the development of associate degree programs. Practical nursing programs would need to be replaced with programs for beginning technical nursing practice in junior and community colleges.

1966–1968 Negative response to the position statement is overwhelming. An important consideration contributing to the reaction is that in 1966, 85.8 percent of employed registered nurses are graduates of diploma programs and have not progressed beyond that level of education (American Nurses' Association, 1971, p. 10). The ANA position paper does receive support from nurse educators in the academic arena and the Conference of Catholic Schools of Nursing (Fondiller, 1980).

After publication of the 1965 position paper, a newly appointed ANA Commission on Nursing Education turns its attention to continuing education. It identifies a framework for future projects, which are to include: (1) enunciating the purposes and characteristics of education for nurses; (2) proposing a total system of formal education in nursing; (3) developing guidelines for community planning for nursing education, and (4) identifying inadequacies in the existing system of education and health care, and nursing education's involvement in that area (American Nurses' Association, 1968, p. 11).

May 1969   The ANA Commission on Nursing Education sends letters of communication to state nurses' associations and state boards to reemphasize the importance of planned educational systems specific to each area (Fondiller, 1980, p. 65).

1973   Eight years after ANA's forthright position on entry into practice, the Commission on Nursing Education takes what many view as a compromise of the association's earlier position by acknowledging diploma schools of nursing and their graduates. The "Statement on Graduates of Diploma Schools of Nursing" asserts: "Neither license or formal education credentials are measures of the quality of a nurse's practice, nor is the professional label such a measure, although they are often so misused" (American Nurses' Association, 1973).

1978   At the 1978 ANA convention, the Commission on Nursing Education introduces new resolutions on entry into practice. Three resolutions are adopted:

1. That ANA ensure two categories of nursing practice to be identified and titled by 1980, that by 1985, the minimum preparation for entry into professional nursing practice be the baccalaureate in nursing, that ANA work with state and other nurses' associations to identify and define two categories of nursing practice, and that national guidelines for implementation be identified and reported back to ANA by 1980;
2. That ANA establish a mechanism for deriving a comprehensive statement of competencies for the two categories of nursing practice by 1980;
3. That ANA actively support increased accessibility to high quality career mobility programs that utilize flexible approaches for individuals seeking academic degrees in nursing [American Nurses' Association, 1978].

It is difficult without detailed examination to determine what is new in these resolutions in comparison to the 1965 resolutions. Two explicit deadlines are added: 1980 for naming and describing two categories of nursing practice, and 1985 for implementing them. Implicit in the 1978 resolutions is the need to differentiate credentialing for the baccalaureate and the less-than-baccalaureate-prepared nurse. There are no specifics as to how this differentiation would occur—whether it would be licensing, certification, or another method.

Another change in the resolution involves terminology. The term *level* was rejected and *category* substituted—perhaps to provide a more neutral flavor. The term *professional* is specified for one category of nurse, and the other category is left untitled. However, the requirement of associate degree education for the untitled category is reaffirmed. Perhaps the most striking difference in the 1965 and 1978 position papers is the third resolution legitimizing career mobility.

1980 At the 1980 ANA biennial convention, the House of Delegates, by consensus, delays the decision on titles until 1982, when the ANA's Commission on Education would complete its report offering a comprehensive statement of competencies ("American Nurses' Association Convention," 1980). Further progress seems to be stalled as state associations struggle for consensus. The 1978 ANA State Action Survey had indicated that only eight states took formal positions on entry into practice, and only three, New York, Ohio, and Tennessee, called for two levels of nursing practice, at the associate level and the baccalaureate level ("Entry into Practice Survey," 1978).

1982 At the 1982 ANA biennial convention, delegates are preoccupied with the change from a trilevel membership—local, state, and national—to a federation as state nurses' associations. In the midst of the confusion surrounding its structural change, ANA adopts an amendment to "move forward in the coming biennium, to expedite implementation of the baccalaureate in nursing as the minimum educational qualification for the practitioner in nursing practice." This amendment further clarifies that the baccalaureate is to be the "minimum educational qualification for entry into professional nursing practice" ("ANA Votes Federation," 1982, p. 1251).

1985 Twenty years after ANA issued its historical position statement calling for the baccalaureate degree as the minimum education level for the professional nurse, the ANA House of Delegates pushes the goal closer to reality ("ANA Delegates Vote to Limit RN Title," 1985, p. 1016). The 680-member house voted by a decisive majority that the title "registered nurse" should be reserved for the professional nurse—the BSN graduate. They adopt "associate nurse" as the title for technical nurses and establish the associate degree in nursing from a state-chartered institution as the minimum educational requirement. The associate nurse title is one of 17 proposed for technical nurses at the meeting.

Delegates at the 1985 convention also approve a resolution directing the ANA Board of Directors to develop a national action plan to implement recommendations on education and titling, enlisting the ANA cabinets on nursing education, practice, and service to define the scope of practice at both the technical and professional level. The plan will involve state nurses' associations, the National Council of State Boards of Nursing, individual state boards of nursing, and national licensed practical nursing organizations.

NATIONAL LEAGUE FOR NURSING

1950 The 1950 convention of the National League of Nursing Education, the predecessor of the National League for Nursing, adopts a statement on "Principles Relating to Organization, Control and Administration of Nursing Education," which becomes the basis for the NLN's philosophy of moving nursing education into institutions of higher learning.

1954 The NLN board issues a "Tentative Statement on Nursing Education" (1954) in an attempt to assure support for and understanding of its goals for nursing. The statement recognizes four groups of personnel as essential for nursing service, but states that only three require formal nursing education. Of these three, the first would be skilled in carrying out some of the activities in nursing care; the second is skilled in carrying out broad and complex activities in nursing care; and the third category is prepared for highly complex activities in various nursing specialties. Given these categories,

> The goal in nursing education is the improvement of each type of educational program in accordance with the specific objectives of the school to the end that each student who completes a program may render maximum service to the area of nursing for which she is prepared. . . . Advancement from one type of educational program in nursing to another type will require careful study of current practices by representatives of the various types of institutions preparing nurses, with an open-mindedness on the part of all concerned [p. 83].

Educators' reactions are conflicting because of the need to fit the products of four educational programs into three categories of personnel.

1961 NLN publishes *Nursing Education Programs Today*. The publication deals little with future goals; rather it delineates nursing education as it exists and reiterates the organization's support of four types of nursing programs.

1965 The NLN convention offers NLN's first definitive stand on the future goals of nursing education. Based largely on the publication *Perspectives for Nursing* (National League for Nursing, 1965), NLN members adopt what would become known as Resolution No. 5:

> The National League for Nursing in convention assembled recognizes and strongly supports the trend toward college-based programs of nursing. The National League for Nursing recommends community planning which will recognize the need for immediate expedition of recruitment efforts which will increase the number of applicants to these programs and implement the orderly movement of nursing education into institutions of higher education in such a way that the flow of nurses into the community will not be interrupted.
>
> To forward the continuing professionalization of nursing reflected in this statement, the National League for Nursing shall sponsor a vigorous campaign of interpreting the different kinds of initial preparation for personnel prepared to perform complementary but different functions.
>
> The National League for Nursing strongly endorses educational planning for nursing at local, state, regional, and national levels to the end that through an orderly development, a desirable balance of nursing personnel with various kinds of preparation become available to meet the nursing needs of the nation and to insure the uninterrupted flow of nurses into the community ["National League for Nursing 1965 Convention," p. 36].

During the years that follow, NLN will attempt to deal with negative response to Resolution No. 5.

1967 The NLN Board of Directors endorses the "Statement on Nursing Education," which reaffirms the resolution. It encourages community planning for educational change and the development of accredited quality baccalaureate and associate degree programs (Fondiller, 1980). NLN emphasizes its role in consultation and accreditation services to meet that end.

1967 At the NLN convention, efforts to rescind Resolution No. 5 fail. The convention approves a restructuring that establishes a Division for Agency Members, which consists of five nursing education councils and two nursing service councils.

As a result of contention from the League's Council of Diploma Programs, the NLN Board of Directors subsequently withdrew the 1967 "Statement on Nursing Education" in the belief that it did not reflect League's entire position (Fondiller, 1980, pp. 103–104).

1972 The NLN Board of Directors approves the statement "Nursing Education in the Seventies," which asks all educational institutions "to make a substantive reappraisal of their current approaches and respond appropriately in view of the needs of society for nursing personnel in the seventies and beyond" (National League for Nursing, 1972).

February 1981 The NLN Board of Directors again affirms its support for all programs in its "Position Statement on Preparation for Practice in Nursing (National League for Nursing, 1981). It cites the "social reality" of different types of individuals seeking careers in nursing as its rationale.

February 1982 The NLN Board of Directors issues a new position statement naming the baccalaureate degree as the minimum preparation for professional nursing practice. It further states:

> Nursing, as an occupation, in the broadest sense, covers a wide range of activities that may be viewed as a continuum beginning with simple nurturing tasks, progressing through increasingly complex responsibilities, and culminating in critical decision-making activities. To meet the reality of this wide range of responsibilities and activities, a corresponding range of nursing practice roles is required; these have come to be referred to as vocational, technical, and professional nursing practice. . . .
> Given the need for such a broad background in the arts and sciences, as well as nursing, professional nursing practice requires the minimum of a baccalaureate degree with a major in nursing. Preparation for technical nursing practice requires an associate degree or a diploma in nursing. Preparation for

vocational nursing requires a certificate or diploma in vocational/practical nursing.

Therefore, to meet varied needs of the public, the National League for Nursing supports the education of nurses in programs that differ in purposes and lengths and that prepare for varying kinds of practice entailing different degrees of responsibility [National League for Nursing, 1982].

The statement goes further to support educational mobility and encourage community planning to ensure appropriate personnel to meet the communities' needs.

1983 Conflict over the 1982 position is evident at the NLN biennial convention. Some delegates assert the importance of articulation and educational mobility, while others warn of problems with articulation models and criticize associate degree educators "who prepare students to merely go on to senior colleges, at one extreme, and, at the other, those who offer mini-BSN programs" ("NLN Reaffirms Its BSN Stance," 1983).

1984 In response to concerns expressed by the Council of Associate Degree Programs about misinterpretation of the League's position, the NLN Board of Directors reaffirms its support for the current system of licensure ("Board Highlights," 1984). The goal of the NLN Committee on Long-Range Planning for nursing education is formulated as "To achieve an adequate supply of appropriately prepared nurses through assuring a high quality system of nursing education" ("Anatomy of the NLN of the Future," 1984). No mention is made of the entry issue.

June 1985 At the NLN convention, 16 resolutions are proposed, one of which deals with continued support for associate degree programs to prepare graduates for entry into RN practice, with additional credentialing mechanisms to attest to preparation and competencies of the professional baccalaureate-prepared nurse beyond those now required ("League Prepares to Step Boldly," 1985). However, the resolution was tabled because of concern over how it would be implemented.

October 1985 The NLN Board of Directors takes definitive action on the education issue, passing the following motion:

NLN supports two levels of nursing practice, professional and associate. Further, the NLN supports the councils working closely with the ANA cabinets to help define the scope and practice of nurses within these levels ["Board Supports Move to Two Levels," 1985].

The League's president, Jacquelyn Kinder (1985) urges constituents to see the action as a "call for unity and a firm effort to place NLN at the center of the educational debate in order to ensure a voice for [its] constituencies." The reasoning behind the board's position is twofold: first, to prepare nurses for more independence and accountability in a changing health care delivery system, and second, to involve all constituents in an implementation plan. Kinder's message stresses that the action "represents the statement of a goal to be worked toward. The mechanisms and strategies to implement this goal are not yet determined."

CURRENT ANA AND NLN POSITIONS

January 1986   The NLN council chairs meet with the ANA cabinet heads at the League headquarters in New York City to discuss the respective positions of the two organizations on titling and licensure, to identify areas of agreement and issues requiring further exploration and resolution, and to begin to consider plans for implementation of two levels of nursing practice. This is the first time since the two major national nursing organizations were founded that representatives have met to discuss the entry-into-practice issue. Areas of consensus are: (1) that there should be two levels of nursing practice, a professional and an associate level, that nursing education should take place in accredited institutions of higher learning; (2) that the second level is the associate level, for which one would be prepared in an associate degree program in nursing; (3) that the first level is the professional level, for which one would be prepared in a baccalaureate program in nursing; (4) that the historic roots of nursing education lie in diploma education; and (5) that in the future, diploma programs will integrate or articulate with associate degree or baccalaureate programs. Further discussion centers on scope of practice issues. It is also agreed that the scope of practice of the associate nurse of the future should be no less than the level of competency required of today's associate degree graduate. Issues for further consideration include educational mobility, requirements for currently licensed individuals and the restructuring of the nursing educational system. It is agreed that the two organizations will meet again at the

ANA convention in May of that year ["Historic NLN/ANA Strategic Planning Meeting," 1986].

February 1986   NLN educational and service chairs meet and propose an Intercouncil Task Force (which is later approved by NLN's Board of Directors), to be composed of two representatives from each educational council. The task force's function is to "define guideposts for articulation; identify other mechanisms for validating previous knowledge in addition to challenge examinations, identify barriers to educational mobility, and make recommendations for removing the barriers; and identify activities that encourage and facilitate the articulation process" ("Chairs/Vice Chairs Task Force," 1986). In addition to forming the task force, the chairs and vice chairs also develop the following "Interpretive Statement on NLN Position in Support of Two Levels of Practice," which is approved by the Board of Directors:

> In October 1985, the NLN Board of Directors approved the following motion:
>
> > "NLN supports two levels of nursing practice, professional and associate. Further, NLN supports the councils working closely with ANA cabinets to help define the scope and practice of nurses within these levels."
>
> This position represents a statement of a future goal to be achieved by the membership and the profession.
>
> Accordingly, the intent of this interpretive statement is to set forth the general principles reflecting the values, priorities, and strategies of NLN in working toward the achievement of this goal.

GENERAL PRINCIPLES

- NLN supports the concept of redefined levels of nursing practice, professional and associate, with licensure yet to be stipulated, and a scope of practice for each yet to be established. The professional scope of practice will be greater than the current registered nurse level; the associate scope of practice will be no less than the level required for current graduates of the associate degree program.
- The domain and scope of practice for professional and associate nursing will evolve from continuing assessments of societal needs for health care services, and from

existing and emerging studies of current practice parameters.

- NLN supports a nursing education system that is responsive to demands for nursing personnel.
- NLN will continue to support the universe of nursing education in carrying out its quality assurance program through such mechanisms as accreditation and peer review.
- NLN will provide leadership within nursing education for remapping the education system in order to establish a foundation for successful transition to a two-level structure.
- NLN will pursue activities to align legal and licensing provisions when the scope of practice for professional and associate nurses is defined. The scope of practice to be established for future practitioners will build on current practice and licensure. Future licenses associated with educational credentials should not be lesser in value than licenses associated with current educational levels.
- NLN wishes to respect and preserve the opportunity now available to nurses to qualify for comparable licensure in states other than those in which they were educated and examined.
- NLN wishes to emphasize that the intent of the position is to maximize educational mobility and strengthen educational support for expanding scope of practice.

PRIORITIES AND STRATEGIES

- Maintaining momentum for maximum career and educational mobility.
- Establishing domain and scope of practice for professional and associate levels.
- Planning and implementing regional planning for educational transition.
- Building a community of opinion in support of changes.
- Collaborating with other national nursing organizations in pursuit of goals for improving nursing practice and education [National League for Nursing, 1986].

A regional Action Plan for implementation of the position for two levels of nursing practice is approved in concept at the February NLN Board of Directors meeting ("Activities Related to Two Levels of Practice," 1986). It calls for the establishment of six to ten regional programs in cooperation with colleges, health care delivery systems, and NLN constituent leagues throughout the country to conduct regional programs, workshops, and seminars to promote understanding of the board's position and, through discussion, to obtain information as to how the policy can be equitably and effectively implemented.

OTHER ORGANIZATIONS

Although they are the largest of the nursing organizations, ANA and NLN are not the only nursing associations to take a stand on issues of titling and licensure for nurses. Nor are nursing organizations the only groups whose positions on this issue have an effect on the profession.

A number of national nursing specialty organizations were joined in 1973 into a federation with ANA. Of these groups, the following support the baccalaureate degree as the educational requirement for professional nursing practice:

- American Association of Colleges of Nursing
- American Association of Critical-Care Nurses
- American Association of Nephrology Nurses and Technicians
- American Association of Occupational Health Nurses
- American Public Health Association/Public Health Nurse Division
- American Organization of Nurse Executives
- Association of Operating Room Nurses
- Association of Rehabilitation Nurses
- American Association of Nurse Anesthetists; Council on Accreditation of Nurse Anesthesia Educational Programs/ Schools
- National Association of Pediatric Nurse Associates and Practitioners
- Nurses Association of the American College of Obstetricians and Gynecologists
- Oncology Nursing Society
- Emergency Nurses Association

The National Federation of Licensed Practical Nurses, a federation of state associations organized in 1949 and made up entirely of licensed practical or vocational nurses, also supports the baccalaureate as the minimal educational requirement for professional nursing practice.

The American Association of Colleges of Nursing was established in 1969. It is a national organization exclusively devoted to furthering the goals of college and university schools of nursing. Its membership is over 390 institutions offering baccalaureate and graduate programs. AACN's position on entry into practice was stated in a letter from its president, Linda Amos, to ANA President Eunice Cole (March 31, 1986):

> Baccalaureate nurses are prepared to assume responsibility for nursing and health care primary, secondary, and tertiary systems. As practitioner-generalists, their knowledges and skills are required in all nursing service systems and, as such, should constitute the bulk of the practicing nursing population if sound goals for health care are to be achieved.
>
> This statement relates to one of the major purposes of AACN. We believe that it is congruent with ANA's position to establish the baccalaureate as the minimum educational requirement for licensure to practice professional nursing, and to retain the legal title "Registered Nurse" for the baccalaureate prepared nurse.

The American Organization of Nurse Executives approved a "Position Statement on Educational Preparation for Nursing Practice" at its October 1986 annual meeting. The statement affirmed the organization's position that

> baccalaureate education in nursing should be the basic preparation for professional nursing practice. The AONE recognizes two levels of educational preparation for nursing practice: the baccalaureate degree in nursing and the associate degree in nursing. This position reflects AONE's support for separate licensure processes based on scopes of practice defined by the profession [American Organization of Nurse Executives, 1986].

The statement also recommends the standardization among states of titles for each type of educational preparation to the extent possible. To ensure the adequate provision of nursing care during the necessary transitional period, AONE supports:

- Establishment of a grandfather clause that will ensure continued nursing practice privileges and interstate mobility for registered nurses and practical nurses licensed at the time of transition

- Collaboration between schools and colleges of nursing to provide opportunities to obtain baccalaureate or associate degrees in nursing for RNs and LPNs licensed at the time of transition
- Employment strategies and educational programs designed to facilitate the efforts of individuals seeking to obtain baccalaureate or associate degrees in nursing
- Collaboration between nursing service and nursing education to delineate scopes of practice that respond to patient needs and reflect the two types of educational preparation
- Intensive recruitment of qualified applicants into the profession of nursing

The National Council of State Boards of Nursing is the collective organization of the individual state boards of nursing that are its members. The NCSBN oversees the development of the National Council Licensure Examination (NCLEX) used by all the state boards. In August 1986, the NCSBN Delegate Assembly approved a recommendation that the NCLEX-RN test plan be revised to base it on the outcomes of the council's *Study of Nursing Practice and Role Delineation and Job Analysis of Entry Level Performance of Registered Nurses* (National Council of State Boards of Nursing, 1986). Although a major revision was not recommended, some revision was suggested to bring the current test plan into closer agreement with the practice of entry-level registered nurses as determined by the study.

There are other non-nursing organizations with varied membership that have an effect on professional nurses and the services they provide. The policy statements that these organizations issue on educational requirements for professional nursing practice are important to the success of nursing in settling the critical issue of educational preparation for entry into practice. One such powerful organization is the American Hospital Association. The AHA's most recent statement on nursing education continues to support all forms of nursing education:

The AHA reiterates its support for all three types of programs of nursing education: associate, diploma, and baccalaureate. All three are needed to provide an adequate supply of nurses for hospitals. As a modification to previous position, however, the Association believes that a baccalaureate degree should be an attainable goal for each student and practicing nurse, in or from an associate or diploma program, and provision must be made for crediting their courses and experience toward the baccalaureate degree [American Hospital Association, undated].

AHA reflects these concepts in its *Guidelines on Educational Mobility in Nursing* (American Hospital Association, 1984). AHA believes educational standards are the responsibility of the profession of nursing and of educational institutions. The translation of those educational standards into standards of practice is the responsibility of the state government. AHA further recognizes that the hospital has the primary responsibility to deal with issues of employment and utilization of nurses with different preparations and to develop standards to assure quality of practice within the institution. To meet this responsibility:

1. AHA reaffirms the intent of the *Guidelines on Educational Mobility in Nursing* that efforts should be undertaken to facilitate the concept that a baccalaureate or higher degree in nursing should be an attainable personal goal for each registered nurse and nursing student, in or from an associate or diploma program. AHA will develop an action plan that assists in the implementation of the guidelines.

2. AHA will encourage members to pursue and support sound programs that provide opportunities for prospective students, students, and practicing nurses that facilitate transition between educational programs.

3. AHA will urge state boards of nursing, state boards of higher education, and regional accrediting bodies to work positively with hospital-based nursing education programs in the development of alternative nursing education programs.

4. AHA will continue to assess emerging issues related to nurse education, nurse titling, and licensure from an employer's perspective and will make this assessment an ongoing agenda item.

5. AHA will continue to collect information, assume a clearinghouse function, and provide technical assistance on nurse education, nurse titling, and licensure issues to AHA constituencies and others.

6. AHA will urge state hospital associations to become familiar with their respective state nurse practice acts and implement an educational process about nurse education, nurse titling, and licensure. It will urge that state hospital associations communicate with state boards of nursing about the employer's perspective, nurse education, nurse titling, and related licensure issues, and will initiate with state hospital associations a technical assistance program on nursing education, nurse titling, and licensure issues.

7. AHA will continue to support mechanisms that ensure interstate mobility for nurses.

8. AHA will continue to seek appropriate financial support for nursing educational programs and to aid in the recruitment of potential nurses to the profession.

9. The AHA will rapidly develop an action plan to assist in the implementation of these recommendations [American Hospital Association, 1984].

The American Medical Association, the primary organization for physicians in this country, founded in 1847, has no official statement on the professional requirements for entry into practice for professional nurses. AMA supports all levels of nursing education.

REFERENCES

Activities related to two levels of practice. (1986). *Nursing & Health Care*, 7(4), 177.

American Hospital Association. (1984). *Guidelines on educational mobility in nursing*. Chicago: American Hospital Association.

American Hospital Association. (Undated). *Policy strategy on nurse education, titling and licensure*. Chicago: American Hospital Association.

American Nurses' Association. (1968). *A blueprint to build on: A report to members, 1966–68*. New York: American Nurses' Association.

American Nurses' Association. (1978). *House of Delegates resolutions*. Kansas City, MO: American Nurses' Association.

American Nurses' Association. (1973). *A statement on graduates of diploma schools of nursing*. Kansas City, MO: American Nurses' Association.

American Nurses' Association convention 1980. (1980). *American Journal of Nursing*, 80(7), 132.

American Nurses' Association's first position on education for nursing. (1965). *American Journal of Nursing*, 65(12), 106–111.

American Organization of Nurse Executives. (1986, October). *AONE Position Statement: Educational Preparation for Nursing Practice*. Chicago: American Organization of Nurse Executives.

ANA delegates vote to limit RN title to BSN grad; Associate nurse wins vote for technical title. (1985). *American Journal of Nursing*, 85(9), 1016.

ANA votes federation. (1982). *American Journal of Nursing*, 82, 251.

Anatomy of the NLN of the future—We want your ideas. (1984). *Nursing & Health Care*, 5(7), 367.

Board highlights. (1984). *Nursing & Health Care*, 5(3), 127.

Board supports move to two levels of nursing practice. (1985). *Nursing & Health Care*, 6(10), 521.

Brown, E. L. (1948). *Nursing for the future*. New York: Russell Sage Foundation.

Chairs/vice chairs task force formed. (1986). *Nursing & Health Care, 7*(4), 183.

Entry into practice survey. (1978, April). *American Journal of Nursing, 78*, 535, 566–572.

Fondiller, S. H. (1980). *The entry dilemma: The National League for Nursing and the higher education movement, 1952–1972*. New York: National League for Nursing.

Henson, H. C. (1960). *Supplemental report: Proceedings of the forty-second convention of the American Nurses' Association, May 2–6*. New York: American Nurses' Association.

Historic NLN/ANA strategic planning meeting held. (1986). *Nursing & Health Care, 7*(4), 183.

Kinder, J. (1985). Charting nursing's future (Editorial). *Nursing & Health Care, 6*(10), 519.

League prepares to step boldly into coming biennium. (1985). *Nursing & Health Care, 6*(6), 301–310.

National Commission for the Study of Nursing and Nursing Education. (1970). *An abstract for action*. New York: McGraw-Hill Book Co.

National Council of State Boards of Nursing. (1986). *A Study of Nursing Practice and Role Delineation and Job Analysis of Entry Level Performance of Registered Nurses*. Chicago: National Council of State Boards of Nursing.

National League for Nursing. (1986, February). *Interpretive statement on NLN position in support of two levels of nursing practice*. New York: National League for Nursing.

National League for Nursing. (1972). *Nursing education in the seventies*. New York: National League for Nursing.

National League for Nursing. (1961). *Nursing education programs today*. New York: National League for Nursing.

National League for Nursing. (1965). *Perspectives for nursing*. New York: National League for Nursing.

National League for Nursing. (1982, February). *Position statement on nursing roles—Scope and preparation*. New York: National League for Nursing.

National League for Nursing. (1981, February). *Position statement on preparation for practice in nursing*. New York: National League for Nursing.

National League for Nursing 1965 convention, San Francisco, May 3–7. (1965, June). *Nursing Outlook, 13*, 36–52.

NLN reaffirms its BSN stance despite technical nursing rift. (1983). *American Journal of Nursing, 83*(7), 995.

Tentative statement on nursing education. (1954, February). *Nursing Outlook, 2*, 83–84.

APPENDIX B

State Positions on Titling and Licensure

Sylvia Edge

INTRODUCTION

The practice of nursing by competent persons is necessary for the protection of the public health, safety, and welfare. The identification of the knowledge and skills needed to provide safe and effective nursing care has been delegated to boards of nursing by state legislatures. This tradition dates back to the mandating of the first board of nursing by the North Carolina legislature in 1903. In addition, boards have been authorized to determine if the minimum essential knowledge and skills needed are found in particular candidates for licensure. This *minimum* essential level of competence in nursing is defined as the ability to perform skillfully and proficiently the functions that are within the legally defined role of the licensee, and to demonstrate the interrelationship of essential knowledge, judgment, and skill.

As of August 1986, at least 48 state nurses' associations and 20 nursing and health care organizations have taken positions to change the educational requirements for entry into nursing practice. The most widely recommended change has been to designate baccalaureate degree education in nursing as the requirement for licensure at the professional level and associate degree nursing education as the requirement for licensure at the technical level.

Thus, there would be (1) one entry point for each level of licensure, (2) a need for the boards of nursing to redefine the legal scope of nursing practice.

The table on the following pages summarizes the positions and actions of the state nurses' associations, the individual state boards of nursing, and the resulting legislative actions. The information was current as of August 1986 unless otherwise indicated.

Summary of State Actions on Titling and Licensure*

State	State Nurses' Association Position	Board of Nursing Action	Legislative Action
Alabama	"Resolved: that members of the Alabama State Nurses' Association declare its support of the 1985 resolution that entry level into nursing practice be the Bachelor of Science in Nursing Degree." Alabama Commission on Nursing has established a committee to study issue.	Board has not taken any action but does have a representative on the task force of the commission charged to study the issue. This task force may come up with a statement in early 1987. (Represents RNs and LPNs.)	
Alaska	Position not firmly decided, but leaning toward BSN-RN and ADN-LPN. Statewide committee to develop position—bill to be introduced.		
Arizona	Accepts ANA position.	No position taken.	No legislation pending. Legislative body meets January–May, so they do not anticipate any action prior to 1987.

*Information is as of August 1, 1986, unless otherwise indicated.

131

State	State Nurses' Association Position	Board of Nursing Action	Legislative Action
Arkansas	"Recommendation: that ASNA support ANA position of baccalaureate in nursing as the minimum preparation for entry into professional nursing practice; support inclusion of a position statement that would allow all currently registered nurses, at time of legal passage of the baccalaureate degree as the minimum level of entry into professional nursing, to continue to be licensed with all the rights, privileges, and responsibilities appropriate for professional nursing; support the associate degree in nursing as the appropriate education for technical nursing practice; appoint two subcommittees composed of nurses in education, administration, and clinical practice, and representatives of the overall membership to: (a) develop statements regarding scope of practice, competencies, licensure, and titles for professional nursing and technical nursing practice and (b) coordinate a master plan for implementation of entry into practice."	No position taken.	The state Department of Vocational-Technical Education has proposed legislation for funding a pilot "1 + 1" program that would admit LPNs only and award the ADN after a calendar year's study. The proposed program would be a joint effort between the Vo-Tech system and a selected community college. (The program has not been presented to the board of nursing for approval.)

California	LVN Board—Task force established; final report, May 1986. RN Board—Board has no current plans to take a position.
Colorado	No position taken. (Represents RNs and LPNs.)
Connecticut	CSNA supports ANA position and has a committee working on strategies.	No current legislation pending. Board gave testimony this year to CSNA recommending status quo—i.e., no change in entry. (Represents RNs and LPNs.)
Delaware	No formal position to date. Remain at a "membership information" level as issue is still volatile.	No position taken to date.
District of Columbia		This issue is not a priority at this time. RNs in DC are working for passage of revised Nurse Practice Act.
Florida	"Resolved: that Deans and Directors of Nursing Programs in Florida continue to support the offering of a variety of routes to prepare students for initial licensure; that a national examination for minimal safe practice be administered to all graduates eligible for initial licensure as a	No position taken. (Represents RNs and LPNs.)

133

State	State Nurses' Association Position	Board of Nursing Action	Legislative Action
	registered nurse; that an additional examination be developed to test the discrete competencies of the graduates with baccalaureate and generic higher degrees in nursing; that individuals who successfully pass the basic national examination be titled and registered nurse technologist (RNT); that individuals who successfully pass the baccalaureate competency examination be titled and registered professional nurse (RNP)." Adopted by FNA House of Delegates 10/3/84. The deans and directors are meeting with directors of nursing service to collaborate on the expectations of new graduates of each program and to develop guidelines on how the graduates are used differently in practice.		
Georgia	"Resolved: (1) that the Georgia Nurses' Association will work toward making the baccalaureate degree the basic level of preparation for new professional nurses in Georgia by the year 1990; (2)	The board of nursing is encouraging educational mobility for licensed practical nurses to become registered nurses. No legislation is planned to address entry level for registered nurses.	

134

that the Georgia Nurses' Association work with the Georgia Board of Nursing, the National Association of State Boards, and the American Nurses' Association to develop two state board examinations for two clearly defined and titled levels of nursing practice; (3) that the Georgia Nurses' Association work with the Georgia Hospital Association, Medical Association of Georgia, University System of Georgia Board of Regents, the Licensed Practical Nurses Associations, and other nursing organizations in developing a mechanism to ensure utilization of the two levels of nursing practice within standards of practice developed by the American Nurses' Association; (4) that the Georgia Nurses' Association work with the University System of Georgia Board of Regents, private colleges and universities in efforts to develop new baccalaureate nursing programs in areas where none presently exist; (5) that the Georgia Nurses' Association continue to support and promote the GNA Southern Performance Assessment Center

There were no plans to introduce a new Practice Act in the 1986 General Assembly.

The Georgia Department of Education Office of Vocational Education has filed a "letter of intent" with the Georgia Board of Nursing that a proposal will be developed and submitted for approval of an LPN/RN Career Mobility Education Program jointly sponsored by Athens Area Vocational Technical School and the University of Georgia.

State	State Nurses' Association Position	Board of Nursing Action	Legislative Action
	Activities as one alternative to generic education; (6) that GNA oppose the awarding of an associate degree by practical nursing programs in vocational schools and strongly support the Georgia Board of Nursing in maintaining the quality of patient care by ensuring that candidates for licensure as registered nurses are graduates of currently approved professional nursing programs."		
Hawaii		No position taken. (Represents RNs and LPNs.)	
Idaho		Board is developing position statement.	
Illinois	Supports ANA position.	Proposed Model Nurse Practice Act, Draft 3, deleted the word "practical" and substituted the word "associate," implying a change in name only. The scope of practice for this associate nurse is essentially the same scope of practice that has been defined for the practical nurse. Draft 6 of this Proposed Model is now available. (11/7/86)	Plan to introduce legislation in 1987.

| Indiana | | Board supports all levels of practice authorized by statute. | |
| Iowa | At the 1985 INA conference, a proposal was presented that there be two educational preparation levels for entry into nursing practice: PN and RN with AD for PN and BS for RN. Task force established with a goal of finding common goal by 1990. | In the 1985 Iowa Legislative session, Senate File 432 was introduced to change the composition of the Iowa Board of Nursing but was not passed. The current law requires the Board composition to be one registered nurse representing the colleges and universities, one registered nurse representing the hospital diploma programs of nursing, one registered nurse representing the area community and vocational technical nursing institutions, one registered nurse practitioner, one licensed practical nurse actively engaged in practice, and two members not registered nurses or licensed practical nurses who shall represent the general public. There has been pressure on the Iowa Board of Nursing to become involved in the resolution of the educational requirements for entry into practice. The Iowa Board of Nursing has requested position statements from the various nursing educational levels but has not taken a position. | See under "Board of Nursing Action." |

State	State Nurses' Association Position	Board of Nursing Action	Legislative Action
Kansas		No position taken. (Represents RNs and LPNs.)	
Kentucky	"Resolved: That the Kentucky Nurses' Association continue efforts to introduce legislation in the 1986 General Assembly to standardize and elevate the education level for future practitioners of nursing; that in 1990, and thereafter, the registered nurse applicant be required to have a baccalaureate degree in nursing; that in 1990, and thereafter, the associate nurse applicant be required to have an associate degree in nursing; that the two present licensure examinations be revised to reflect the minimal competencies required of the registered nurse and associate nurse; that currently licensed nurses be encouraged to increase their knowledge and competency base through continuing education or formal education; that schools of nursing be encouraged to facilitate nurses' attainment of academic degrees; that effective 1990, all nurses	No position taken. (Represents RNs and LPNs.)	Supporters of entry-level changes were dealt a setback when they failed to introduce a bill for the change in the 1986 legislative session, as planned.

then licensed as registered nurses by the Commonwealth of Kentucky will continue to be licensed as registered nurses, regardless of educational preparation; that effective 1990, all nurses then licensed as licensed practical nurses by the Commonwealth of Kentucky will be licensed as associate nurses, regardless of educational preparation." KNA Resolution, 10/85.

Louisiana

The Louisiana State Board of Nursing (LSBN) adopted a motion that entry level into professional nursing practice be at the baccalaureate level. The board approved a recommendation to invite the Louisiana State Board of Practical Nurse Examiners to membership on LSBN's Advisory Council and reaffirmed that graduates of external degree programs are not eligible for licensure in Louisiana by examination or endorsement. The board has placed a moratorium on the establishment of new undergraduate programs in nursing. (This does not preclude restructuring of existing programs.)

The Louisiana State Board of

State	State Nurses' Association Position	Board of Nursing Action	Legislative Action
		Practical Nurse Examiners was not planning to present any legislation in 1986. It is currently undergoing sunset review.	
Maine	Supports the ANA position.	See under "Legislative Action."	The legislature has passed a rather complicated bill revising the nursing practice act, which could implement recommended changes in entry level in 1995, but only if a state commission to be established in the interim finds that a number of stringent conditions have been met. The commission, which includes representatives from a number of organizations strongly opposed to the entry-level changes, must find that, by 1990, the following conditions exist: provisions for no loss of credit for AD graduates going back for a BSN; development of a valid method for assessing the knowledge of nurses (for those returning to school); an adequate number of BSN programs in the state. The commission would also need to conclude, for the change to go forward, that the change would

not have a damaging impact on reciprocity (endorsement) or on the supply of nurses. The legislature is required to vote again on the issue in 1990.

The act states: ". . . All applicants for professional nursing licensure must have completed an approved baccalaureate or graduate degree program in nursing. . . . All applicants for license as a practical nurse must have completed an approved associate degree program in nursing."
Both statements become effective in 1995.

Maryland

Supports ANA position.

The board of examiners of nurses is working on a plan for the implementation of a baccalaureate certification examination. The work is progressing slowly and carefully to ensure that the nursing community is fully informed. The board is presently involved in the development of the competencies and evaluation of the requirements needed to implement such an examination. No final decisions have been made.

State	State Nurses' Association Position	Board of Nursing Action	Legislative Action
Massachusetts	Change in Nurse Practice Act drafted 10/1/84. Proposes two levels of practice: professional nursing (graduate of baccalaureate or higher degree program in nursing) and practical nursing (graduate of associate degree school of nursing). Blueprint calls for (1) filing of this bill in September 1985 with completion date November 1985, (2) filing legislation the first Wednesday in December 1985, (3) developing and implementing network in MNA districts. (1/86)	Maintain current requirements.	
Michigan	Supports the ANA position.	No position taken to date.	
Minnesota	"By 1990 a baccalaureate degree . . . will be the preparation for entry into professional nursing. . . . "Registered Nurses: Education and Practice. The minimal education preparation for entry into professional nursing practice is the baccalaureate degree with a major in nursing. . . . The practice of professional nursing by Registered Nurses occurs within	No position taken.	

142

a variety of settings (primary, secondary and tertiary), in complex and unpredictable situations and is concerned with promoting healthy behaviors as well as providing care for the ill. . . . . The Registered Nurse works directly and indirectly with the assistant to the professional nurse to provide care for individuals and families.

"Assistants to the Professional Nurse: Education and Practice. Assistants to the professional nurse are educated in educational settings by professional nurses. This education prepares the assistant to the professional nurse to perform specific delegated functions. Assistants to the professional nurse have a role in health care only under the direction of a professional nurse. The educational setting for the assistant to the professional nurse shall be the vocational/technical institution and/or the community college." Position statement of MNA, 1985.

State	State Nurses' Association Position	Board of Nursing Action	Legislative Action
Mississippi	"Resolved: that MNA cooperate with the council of deans and directors to collect and analyze data concerning nursing education needs in the state; that MNA encourage the Board of Trustees of State Institutions of Higher Learning to utilize this data in planning and reviewing nursing education programs in the state." A task force has been designated to prepare a position paper for entry into practice. This paper was to be presented to a special session of the House of Delegates in May 1985. The position is that the bachelor's degree will be the minimum preparation for the professional registered nurse.	There are no plans to initiate any new programs or to phase out any existing practical nursing programs. Vocational education serves the entire state of Mississippi by offering practical nursing education in 12 junior college districts. Programs and curricula are being adjusted to meet the needs of employers. The practical nursing education curriculum will be comprehensive and include more emphasis on long-term care needs and communitywide nursing needs. The licensed practical nurse is expected to have increased responsibilities.	
Missouri	Supports ANA position and has formed a task force to study the issue. The Board of Nursing is represented on this task force.	No formal position taken at this time.	
Montana	Will introduce legislation in 1987 requiring baccalaureate for RNs and associate degree for LPNs entering practice in 1992.	Montana attorney general ruled in 1985 that the board cannot change educational rules and regulations.	

State			
Nebraska	Accepts ANA position.	No position taken.	
Nevada		Accepts ANA position with no Level 2 title (ANA title Associate Nurse).	
New Hampshire		No position taken to date.	
New Jersey	NJSNA task force has been meeting to study and determine how to implement the ANA position.	No position taken to date.	
New Mexico		No position taken.	The New Mexico Legislature passed a Senate Joint Memorial requesting the legislature "to direct the board of nursing to create a volunteer task force to develop a comprehensive nursing education plan."
New York	NYSNA supports ANA position and has formulated legislation to effect BSN-RN, and ADN-PN, with reduced scope of practice. This bill is not yet out of committee, but another attempt is expected in the 1987 legislative session.	Accepts ANA position, no titles identified.	See under "State Nurses' Associations."
North Carolina		"In view of recent national activities regarding Entry Into Prac-	No legislative activity planned by the board of nursing.

State	State Nurses' Association Position	Board of Nursing Action	Legislative Action
		tice, the North Carolina Board of Nursing has explored the role and responsibility it has in relationship to the issue. It is important to share our perspective of the scope of the issue, including the potential impact on the public in North Carolina. "The board identified the need for extensive communication among a wide variety of groups prior to engaging in any formal action which might result in alteration or revision of entry level requirements or titling. Review of action taken in other states reveals the need for a major portion of the work effort to focus on delineation of scope of practice and role functions. "The Board believes that there should be two levels of nursing practice. The Board further believes that these two levels must realistically reflect nursing practice. Definition of the scope of practice would have significant impact on curricula of all levels of nursing education. It is of pri-	

mary importance that curricular design be consistent with and reflect the scope of practice. As scope of practice evolves, the validity and reliability of the licensure examination must be evaluated.

"The Board supports the concept of grandfathering; however, implementation becomes quite complex when considered in conjunction with potential change in scope of practice and educational preparation. To assure competency in nursing practice, these aspects must be thoroughly examined and clarified before any definitive statements regarding grandfathering can be made.

"Not only are all of the above factors important to pursue in any deliberation on Entry Into Practice, but consideration must be given to health policies and health care trends. Such factors as patient acuity, advanced technology, and changing practice settings will influence these deliberations.

"The Board firmly believes that there must be collaboration as

147

State	State Nurses' Association Position	Board of Nursing Action	Legislative Action
		the nursing community in North Carolina addresses this issue. Facilitating this collaboration among the many groups affected is the responsibility of the Board.	
		"Multiple strategies will be employed to involve individuals and groups with potential for small group sessions, regional forums, and other forms of communication with the Board as well as other nursing colleagues. It is important for those individuals and groups who wish to participate in these activities to notify the Board.	
		"While the Board does not intend to accept membership on any specific committee, the Board will respond in a consulting capacity. The Board will continue to function in a resource role on legal issues in nursing." North Carolina Board of Nursing Positive Statement on Entry into Practice, 2/86.	

148

| North Dakota | Accepts ANA position. | In January 1986, the North Dakota Board of Nursing promulgated administrative rules that will require, among other changes, nursing education programs to offer specific curriculums leading to the associate degree for practical nurse programs and the baccalaureate degree for registered nurse programs in order to be approved by the board of nursing, effective January 1, 1987. The rules were submitted to the attorney general for his review as required by the Administrative Practices Act. The attorney general approved the rules "as to their legality," and the board officially adopted them on January 16, 1986. The rules were published in the Administrative Code Supplement, March 1986 edition, and have an effective date of March 1, 1986, except for the portion of the rules that were postdated to January 1, 1987. | A hearing was held April 15, 1986, in Williston, North Dakota, regarding the restraining order by two hospitals. On April 24, |

State	State Nurses' Association Position	Board of Nursing Action	Legislative Action
		plaintiffs filed a motion to halt all proceedings and to ask the court to certify two questions of law to the North Dakota Supreme Court, which the District Court accepted over the board's objections. The earliest possible action on the order was expected in Fall 1986.	
		It is the board's belief that the promulgation of these administrative rules is the fulfillment of the North Dakota legislature's mandate as expressed in the North Dakota statutes: "It is essential to govern qualifications for licensure with requirements for the maintenance of high standards."	
Ohio	Supports ANA position.	No position taken to date.	
Oklahoma	Supports ANA position with a different Level 2 title.	Will not take a position. (Represents RNs and LPNs.)	
Oregon	Passed a resolution in April 1985 agreeing to support the "current consensus which exists for two categories of nursing personnel," but stressing that "ONA's	No position to date.	The Oregon Legislative Assembly in its 1985 Session, passed House Bill 2928, sponsored by the Committee on Education, which read in part:

commitment to the future remains the baccalaureate in nursing as the minimal educational preparation for entry into practice."

"(1) In carrying out its duties under ORS 678.150 (6), (7) and (8) the Oregon State Board of Nursing shall not make changes in entry level nursing education or licensure requirements after the effective date of this 1985 Act unless such changes are enacted by the Legislative Assembly.

"(2) In carrying out its duties under ORS 678.150 (7) (j) the Oregon State Board of Nursing shall not prescribe any standard that would substantially alter the practices followed prior to July 1, 1979, in long-term care facilities relating to the administration of noninjectable medication by nursing assistants, except for the training requirements in ORS 678.440."

Pennsylvania

Supports ANA position; has not developed position statement.

"• The Board takes no position on proposed legislative changes to entry level into nursing.

"• The topic is not included in the long range plans of the Board.

State	State Nurses' Association Position	Board of Nursing Action	Legislative Action
		".• The Board supports LPN, Diploma, Associate Degree and Baccalaureate Degree Programs as described in the Rules and Regulations and in accordance with the current law." Pennsylvania Board of Nursing memorandum, 10/86.	
Rhode Island	No position taken.	No position taken.	
South Carolina		The state board of nursing has addressed entry into practice for the past seven years through its advisory committee, the State-wide Master Planning Committee for Nursing Education (SWMPCNE). This committee has developed competencies for two levels of nurses and gone on record as supporting two educational tracks leading to two licensure levels: associate degree for the basic (technical) level and baccalaureate for the advanced (professional) level. The target date for implementation for this proposed plan is 1995. Recommendations include:	

"1. By the year 1995, the minimum educational requirement for entry to practice in South Carolina will be an Associate Degree for technical practice and a Baccalaureate Degree for professional practice. All students enrolled in nursing education programs in 1993 will be in one of the above degree granting programs.

"2. In 1986–1988 open hearings be conducted by the SWMPCNE, State Board of Nursing and CHE to discuss the implementation of the recommendation.

"3. By 1988, a plan be developed to facilitate grandfathering of presently licensed nurses.

"4. That all nursing education programs begin to evaluate their curricula in relationship to the competency study. Results should be communicated to the Statewide Master Planning Committee by the State Board of Nursing which reviews basic programs and by the directors of graduate education programs.

State	State Nurses' Association Position	Board of Nursing Action	Legislative Action
		"5. Emphasis be placed on developing demand data to accurately reflect mix and that this data be required prior to approval of new programs."	
South Dakota		Accepts ANA position, titles not determined.	
Tennessee	Proposed changes in the Nurse Practice Act presented by the Tennessee Board of Nursing in conjunction with the Tennessee Nurses' Association Task Force on the Tennessee Nurse Practice Act propose either statutory or regulatory language for BSN entry for 1991 (professional nurse). Technical nurse means a person licensed by the Tennessee Board of Nursing to practice technical nursing. The TNA has issued a draft of its proposed entry-level bill to be introduced in the legislature in 1987. Beginning in 1991, applicants for licensure as registered nurses would be required to have a BSN. Applicants for licensure as associate nurses	The Tennessee Board of Nursing has appointed a task force on the nurse practice act. Major issues to be considered include: expanded role of the nurse, disciplinary penalties and fines, educational preparation for nursing practice and titling. In December 1986 the Board of Nursing will consider taking a position on level of entry into practice.	

State			
	("licensed to practice technical nursing") would be required to have an ADN.		
Texas	TNA supports work of education committee: RN licensure for both levels with an additional credentialing exam to test for additional competencies of the BSN. (5/85)	No position taken. (Separate RN and LPN boards.)	
Utah	No position taken.		The Utah legislature passed by overwhelming vote and the governor signed on March 17, 1986 legislation denying the State Board of Nursing the power to refuse access to licensure to graduates of accredited schools of nursing. Essentially, the purpose of the law is to make it impossible for the State Board to enact an entry-level measure without going through the legislature. A coalition of ADN and LPN groups and individuals led support for the measure, along with groups representing health care consumers.
Vermont	Accepts ANA position; no titles identified.	No position taken.	

State	State Nurses' Association Position	Board of Nursing Action	Legislative Action
Virginia	"Resolved: that the Virginia Nurses' Association support the premise that the minimum preparation for the professional practice of nursing is the baccalaureate degree in nursing; that VNA implement activities to define entry level competencies for the professional practice of nursing." VNA plans hearings to be held throughout the state on issue of educational preparation, proposed and accepted work of deans of colleges and universities and program heads of community colleges to move toward articulation strategy development.	The Virginia Board of Nursing has completed a comprehensive review of its regulations. Reports are being considered by the Governor's Regulatory Reform Advisory Board. The secondary state-approved vocational practical nursing programs are managed by local school divisions and offer high school seniors and adults an opportunity to enter the labor market as licensed practical nurses. No new secondary programs are planned; phasing out of any of the existing 40+ programs is not planned.	
Virgin Islands		Board is developing position statement.	
Washington	Supports ANA position.	"Resolved: "1. There be a planned phasing out of all PN programs. "2. No new associate degree program established. "3. Baccalaureate programs con-	

156

tinue to accelerate their commitment to increasing the accessibility of baccalaureate education for registered nurses.

"4. Associate degree nursing programs continue to accelerate the availability and accessibility of associate degree education for graduates of college-based and vocational-technical-based practical nurse programs." Motions of the Council on Nursing Education, 4/86.

A bill that would have given the state board of nursing the power to change the educational requirement for licensure has died in committee.

State			
West Virginia	The board of examiners for registered nurses supports the ANA position paper calling for two levels of nursing practice and is studying the issue. No Level 2 title. (Separate RN and LPN boards.)	Board will not take a position. Task force is being formed to address the issue.	
Wisconsin	Nursing Study Committee formulated 14 recommendations, including the following: • Entering practitioners be prepared to meet specified competencies based upon societal and consumer needs for two new entry levels (Level 1 and Level 2) of nursing practice that: (1)		

State	State Nurses' Association Position	Board of Nursing Action	Legislative Action
	share a core of knowledge and skills, and (2) are clearly distinct in terms of accountability and scope of practice. • Educational preparation for entry level nurses incorporate the strengths of the four current programs (PN, ADN, Diploma, BSN) into two new programs (ADN and BSN, revised to meet the specified competencies) without decreasing the number of state and regional graduates. • Any future change in licensure/credentialing laws for nurses be enacted with a "grandfather" clause, stating that new requirements are applicable only to those seeking initial licensure/credentialing after the enactment date, and that already licensed nurses will maintain, at a minimum, their current practice privileges. • Continuing competency of practicing nurses be assured. • Continuing education for nurses be voluntary.		

- ADN and BSN completion programs that adequately and appropriately recognize prior learning be accessible.
- Sufficient numbers of entry-level nurses be prepared to meet the identified statewide need for nurses in all health care delivery settings, especially long-term care.
- Nursing leadership be strengthened by the preparation of sufficient numbers of nurses at the graduate level to meet the identified future needs for teachers, administrators, nurse practitioners, and clinical specialists, and by the provision of relevant continuing education offerings for nurses currently functioning in these roles.

Wyoming

Community college group attempted unsuccessfully to delete the nursing board's authority to approve educational programs. Board plans to develop position statement.